THE NO BS GUIDE FOR CAREGIVERS

How to Survive the Healthcare Maze

Tiffany Auvil, MBA, RN

THE NO BS GUIDE FOR CAREGIVERS How to Survive the Healthcare Maze

ISBN (paperback): 979-8-9960882-0-1

First Edition, June 13, 2026

Independently published Parsons, West Virginia

Cover design by Tiffany Auvil

Edited by Tiffany Auvil

Disclaimer

This book is based on the author's personal experience as a family caregiver and her professional background as a registered nurse and healthcare leader. It is intended as a general guide for navigating the healthcare system and is not a substitute for individualized medical, legal, financial, or professional advice.

The information in this book reflects the author's understanding of the U.S. healthcare system at the time of publication. Healthcare laws, insurance practices, Medicare and Medicaid rules, and clinical guidelines change over time. Always consult qualified professionals — a licensed physician, attorney, financial advisor, or insurance specialist — before making decisions about your or a loved one's care, finances, or legal arrangements.

The author specifically disclaims any responsibility for any liability, loss, or risk, personal or otherwise, that is incurred as a consequence, directly or indirectly, of the use or application of any of the contents of this book.

Names and identifying details of some individuals mentioned in this book may have been changed to protect privacy. The author's late husband, Dave, appears under his real name.

If you or someone you love is in a mental health crisis, please call or text 988. If you are experiencing a medical emergency, call 911.

A Note on AI Assistance

This book was drafted with the help of generative AI tools used to structure, organize, and refine the content. All personal experiences, professional expertise, editorial choices, and final wording are the author's own. The AI helped shape the book; the story, knowledge, and heart of it are hers.

Contents

For all the caregivers who struggle daily...

I see you. You are not alone.

Chapter One

Introduction

Start Here. Breathe.

If you picked up this book, something is happening. Maybe your mom just got diagnosed with something you can't pronounce. Maybe your dad fell, and the hospital is talking about "placement" like he's a piece of furniture. Maybe your spouse is sicker than anyone wants to say out loud, and you're the one expected to figure it all out — the appointments, the medications, the insurance, the bills that look like ransom notes.

You are not failing. You are not crazy. You are up against a system that was not built for the people who need it most.

This book is going to walk you through it. Not the polished, motivational version. The real one.

Who I Am, and Why I Wrote This

I'm a registered nurse. I've worked in healthcare leadership long enough to see how the sausage gets made — the rounds, the rushed handoffs, the insurance denials, the discharges that happen before anyone is actually ready, the bills that arrive months later for things you didn't even know happened. I know the inside of this machine.

And then I became a caregiver.

I didn't start out as a nurse. I started out as a volunteer firefighter.

It was 2002. I joined the local volunteer fire department, picked up first aid and CPR, and somewhere in there caught the bug. One thing led to another — EMT certification, then CNA, then an LPN program thirty minutes from home. I'd actually wanted to be a paramedic. I loved the adrenaline, the EMS work, the feeling of being in the middle of something that mattered. But the paramedic program was an hour and a half away, was two years long and cost more than I had. The LPN program was $3,400 and I'd be done in less than a year, making more than a paramedic on the other side of it. So nursing it was — not because it was my dream, but because it made sense.

I never expected to love it. I did.

I worked my way up through the system over the next two decades. Night shift on a med-surg telemetry unit. A GI clinic I hated. Family practice, which I loved. Lead LPN. Population health manager. Nurse manager. And eventually, System Director of Outpatient Clinics for a three-hospital health system spanning four counties. I had done prior authorizations. I had worked with insurance companies. I understood coding and billing and the things that happen behind the scenes that most patients never see. I knew where the red tape lived and how to cut through it.

I knew this system.

In 2016, my husband was diagnosed with stage three renal cell carcinoma. The tumor had been growing on his left kidney for years — slow and quiet — before we caught it. We were lucky. A robotic nephrectomy, one night in the hospital, and he was home the next day. He stayed cancer free for years. We exhaled.

Then, in the fall of 2022, he started having vision problems.

We pushed for answers. An ophthalmologist told him his eyes were fine. They weren't fine. In January 2023, we did a CT — head, chest, abdomen — because in the back of both our minds was the word we didn't want to say out loud: recurrence. The scan confirmed it. His renal cell cancer was back. This time in his pancreas and his liver.

We fought. He fought. And we still couldn't explain the vision.

For months, we assumed it was the renal cell cancer — that it had spread to his eye. That's what made the most sense given his history. It wasn't until January 2024, after a Gamma Knife procedure on what we believed was renal cell metastasis, that the real answer came — violently. He developed severe brain swelling. He needed a craniotomy. Two weeks later, the biopsy results came back. What they found wasn't renal cell cancer at all.

It was lymphoma. Specifically, Central Nervous System Lymphoma — a rare form that stays contained to the brain and spinal cord and almost never shows up anywhere else in the body. What had been in his eye all along was intraocular lymphoma. Not a met. A completely separate cancer. A cancer that if left untreated spreads and becomes Central Nervous System Lymphoma.

I am a registered nurse with over twenty years of experience. I did not know that lymphomas existed that affected only the central nervous system. I had never heard of it. That's not a small thing to admit — and I'm admitting it here on purpose, because if that's true for me, it can be true for anyone, and shame about not knowing something you had no reason to know is a waste of energy you don't have.

He now had two cancers. He fought for another year and four months.

In April 2025, he died at home. With me and our son beside him.

I tell you all of this not for sympathy — though God knows caregiving earns it — but because of what happened in the years between that first scan and that last day. I spent countless hours on the phone with clinics, hospitals, insurance companies. I chased down denials only to find out they weren't real denials.

The night before my husband's first immunotherapy infusion, we got a phone call from the clinic. His insurance had denied the treatment. They couldn't move forward without an authorization.

I knew immediately something was wrong. We had excellent insurance — the kind that didn't even require a prior authorization for an MRI. They were not going to deny immunotherapy. I called the insurance company directly. Spent just a few minutes on the phone with them. They were baffled. They had no record of any denial. As far as they were concerned, there was no issue.

So I went back to the clinic. Multiple calls back and forth. Finally, a nurse read me the CPT code their prior authorization specialist had submitted — the code they'd been trying to get approved for Keytruda.

It was a diagnosis code. Specifically, the diagnosis code for renal cell carcinoma.

The prior authorization specialist had mixed up her codes. She'd submitted a diagnosis code in the field where a CPT code belonged, the system had kicked it back, and somewhere along the line that became "insurance denied it." The night before his first treatment.

I took a breath. I told the nurse — calmly, because none of this was her fault — that she was welcome to pass my cell number along to the prior authorization specialist. And that I would be happy to help her understand the difference between a CPT code and a diagnosis code if she needed the refresher. But that we would be there at 9:30 in the morning.

We were.

His oncologist met us with relief on her face. She told me she was glad I'd pushed, that she always worried when treatments came back denied, but since prior authorizations were handled by a separate department, she'd had no idea the error had even been made. She was finding out the same time we were.

That's the part that stayed with me. The doctor didn't know. The insurance company didn't know. The only person who knew something was wrong — and had the knowledge and the nerve to track down exactly what it was — was me. The caregiver. The one person in that equation with no official role and no authority, just a working knowledge of how the pieces fit together and enough stubbornness to keep making phone calls.

Most people don't have that. Not because they're not smart enough — because no one ever told them this was information they needed to have.

That's what this book is trying to fix.

Here's what surprised me most: even with all my training, even with the badge and the credentials and the years of experience, I still got blindsided. I missed things. I forgot to ask questions I would have nailed a patient's family for not asking. I cried in parking lots. I argued with insurance reps and hung up shaking. I was tired in a way I had never been tired before.

If that happened to me — someone who literally does this for a living — what is happening to everyone else?

That question is why this book exists.

What This Book Will Do

This book is going to give you what nobody handed me when I needed it: a plain-language, no-bullshit guide to caregiving inside the modern healthcare system. We're going to talk about the things healthcare workers don't always explain, either because they don't have time, they assume you already know, or because saying it out loud feels uncomfortable. And yes, some of them they don't even know themselves.

By the time you're done, you'll be able to:

- Walk into appointments knowing what to ask and what to bring.
- Read an insurance denial letter without throwing your phone across the room.
- Tell the difference between a bill and an EOB (and why you shouldn't pay the first thing that arrives).
- Push back without being labeled "that family."
- Recognize when something is genuinely off and what to do about it.
- Take care of yourself enough to keep doing this — because if you fall apart, the whole thing falls apart.

I'm not going to promise you peace. Caregiving doesn't really come with peace, not the kind people post about on Instagram. What I can promise is clarity. You'll know what is happening, why it's happening, and what your next move is.

What This Book Will Not Do

Let me get this out of the way: this is not a feel-good book. It is not going to tell you that everything happens for a reason. It is not going to suggest you light a candle and journal your way out of a Medicare appeal. There are good books out there for the spiritual side of caregiving. This is not one of them.

This book also is not a substitute for medical advice. I'm not your nurse. I'm not your loved one's nurse. I don't know their chart, their meds, or their history. What I can do is teach you how the system thinks, so you can make better decisions inside of it.

And one more thing — I curse sometimes. Not because I'm trying to be edgy, but because that's how I actually talk, and because some of this stuff genuinely calls for it. If that bothers you, this might not be your book. If it's a relief, welcome. You're in the right place.

How to Use This Book

You don't have to read this book front to back. Honestly, you probably don't have time. Caregivers don't sit down with a cup of tea and a highlighter — they read while waiting in pharmacy lines, while the IV pump beeps, at 2 a.m. when they should be sleeping. So I built this book to be skimmable.

Here's how it's organized:

- **Part 1: Foundations.** Getting your feet under you — organizing information, understanding who's who, decoding insurance basics.
- **Part 2: Navigating the System.** Appointments, referrals, urgent care vs ER, hospital stays. The mechanics.
- **Part 3: Advocacy.** How to speak up, when to push, what to do when something feels off.
- **Part 4: Money and Paperwork.** Bills, EOBs, denials, appeals. The boring, expensive stuff that nobody warns you about.
- **Part 5: The Human Side.** The emotional weight, self-care without the bullshit, what happens when treatment stops working, and what comes after.
- **Bonus Section.** Checklists, scripts, worksheets — the stuff you'll actually use.

If something is on fire right now — a denial, a discharge, an appointment tomorrow — flip to that chapter first. Come back to the rest later.

A Few Things to Know Before We Start

Before we go any further, you need to know three things. These aren't warm-up points. They're the whole framework.

- **Healthcare has multiple decision-makers, not one.** Your physician decides what you need medically. The facility decides what it costs and how it's billed. Insurance decides what gets paid. They are not on the same team. They don't always talk to each other. And when they do, they often do not care what the other has to say. You are often the only person who sees all three at once — which is exhausting, and also why your role matters so much.

- **The system is fragmented and not designed for ease.** It was not built around you. It was built around billing codes, productivity metrics, and risk management. That's not a conspiracy theory — it's just how it grew. Once you stop expecting it to be intuitive, things get easier.
- **Caregivers must do three things, constantly: ask questions, track everything, and advocate.** That's the job. Not the job of being a daughter or a son or a spouse — the job of being a caregiver inside this machine. We'll spend the rest of the book turning those three things into specific, doable habits.

A Word About Guilt

I want to say this now, because if I don't, it's going to creep into every chapter. You are going to feel guilty during this. About things you did. Things you didn't do. Things you wished you'd done sooner. Decisions you made with the information you had, that look different now that you have more.

Guilt is not evidence. It's a feeling. It's not a verdict. The fact that you're reading a book to do this better is, by itself, more than most people manage. You are doing your best with a system that is designed in ways that actively make your job harder. When the guilt shows up — and it will — try to remember that.

Do This Next

Before you turn to Chapter 2, do these three things. They take about five minutes total and they'll make everything else in this book easier.

- **Grab a notebook.** Any notebook. A spiral one from the dollar store works fine. Label it with your loved one's name and the year. This is where everything is going to live — phone numbers, appointment notes, questions you want to ask, things doctors said. Don't try to be fancy. Just have one place.
- **Find your loved one's insurance card.** Take a picture of the front and back with your phone. Put it in a folder labeled "Medical" or somewhere you'll find it again. You're going to need this number more times than you can count.
- **Make a short list — five names — of who you can call when this gets hard.** Not who you think you should put on the list. Who would actually answer. Who would actually show up. Keep it short. Keep it real.

That's it. That's day one. We'll build from here.

Take a breath. Turn the page when you're ready.

Chapter Two

Getting Organized From Day One

The Most Boring Chapter That Will Save Your Sanity

I know. The word "organized" makes you want to close this book. You're already drowning, and now I'm going to tell you to make a binder?

Yes. I am.

Here's why: the single biggest predictor of how badly caregiving is going to wreck you is not how sick your person is. It's not the diagnosis. It's whether you can find their information when you need it. Whether you know what medications they're on, who their cardiologist is, what their insurance ID number is, what was said at the appointment last Tuesday.

I have watched smart, competent people fall apart in the ER not because of what was happening to their loved one, but because they couldn't remember if their mom took the blood thinner in the morning or at night. The chaos of not knowing is its own kind of suffering. We're going to fix that today.

The Four Things You Have to Track

There are basically four buckets of information you need to keep on top of: appointments, medications, contacts, and medical history. That's it. Not seven. Not twelve. Four.

If you can keep these four updated — even messily, even imperfectly — you will be ahead of 90% of caregivers walking into appointments today.

1. Appointments

Every appointment, scan, lab, procedure, and follow-up needs to live somewhere you can see it. Not in your head. Not in a stack of paper appointment cards in your purse. Somewhere visible.

Three options that work, in order of how low-tech they are:

- **A paper calendar or planner** — works great if you're not a phone person. Write the date, time, location, doctor's name, and what it's for. Don't trust the appointment card alone. They get lost.
- **A shared digital calendar** — Google Calendar, iCloud, whatever. The advantage: you can share it with siblings or other family members so everyone sees the same thing. This single move can prevent half the family fights you're about to have.
- **A dedicated app** — there are caregiver apps that combine appointments, meds, and notes. They can be useful, but only if you'll actually open them. Don't pay for one if a calendar will do.

Whatever you pick, write down three things for every appointment: the **reason** for the visit, the **address** (offices have multiple locations and you will go to the wrong one), and a **phone number** to call if something goes wrong.

I personally ran a hybrid system. I used a shared google calendar that my husband could also access. I would put the next appointment into the calendar even before we left the check-out window at the clinic. I also wrote the appointment down in the book that I kept all the notes in. I tell you this because you don't have to pick one, you could pick two. Or you could even have something else that works for you. But I do not recommend just allowing the information to live in your head because something will eventually force it out once your brain ends up with too many tabs open.

2. Medications

If you do nothing else this week, make a medication list. Then keep it updated. This single document is going to save your loved one's life one day, and I'm not exaggerating.

A good medication list includes:

- Drug name (both brand and generic, if you know them)
- Dose (e.g., 25 mg)
- How often (twice a day, every morning, etc.)
- What it's for (in plain English — "blood pressure," not "anti-hypertensive")
- Who prescribed it
- Any over-the-counter meds, vitamins, and supplements (these matter — they interact with prescriptions)
- Any herbal supplements or teas your loved one uses — these matter more than most people realize.

A note on that: chamomile can increase bleeding risk and shouldn't be combined with blood thinners. Lavender, skullcap, valerian, and mugwort can all increase sedation and shouldn't be mixed with benzodiazepines. If it goes in the body, it goes on the list.

Print two copies. Put one in your bag. Put one on the fridge. Keep an updated list on the notes app on your phone or in a Google Drive and share it with your loved one and others who may participate in caring for your person. That way if you make updates to the original it will change for everyone else as well. Update it every time something changes. When you go to any appointment — any appointment — you hand over the list. When you go to the ER, you hand over the list before they ask. Half of what goes wrong in healthcare goes wrong because nobody actually knows what someone is taking.

Every appointment, I walked in with two things: a printed copy of his current medication list — drug name, dose, frequency, and the reason he was taking it in plain English — and a notebook where I kept running notes from every visit. Not just his oncology appointments. Ophthalmology too. We spent the better part of that first year bouncing between the two, trying to connect dots that kept not connecting.

I can't tell you how many times his oncologist looked up from the chart and said some version of the same thing: that she didn't worry about my husband the way she worried about some of her other patients. Because she knew I was there. She knew I had it.

That felt good to hear. It also broke my heart a little, every time. Because what it really meant was that the patients who didn't have someone like me — prepared, persistent, fluent in the language — were the ones she did worry about. And there are a lot of them.

A medication list doesn't sound like advocacy. It is. It's the first, most basic form of it. It tells every provider in that room that you are paying attention. That you know what's in your person's body. That if something gets missed, you will catch it. The list itself isn't the point — the message it sends is.

3. Contacts

Every doctor, specialist, pharmacy, home health agency, durable medical equipment company, and case manager who touches your person needs to be in one place. Names, phone numbers, fax numbers (yes, healthcare still uses fax — don't get me started), and what they do.

Here's the format I use, and you can copy it:

Dr. Sarah Chen — Cardiologist — Heartwell Clinic — (555) 123-4567 — fax (555) 123-4570 — last seen 3/14/26 — manages: heart failure meds

That looks like overkill. It is not. Six months from now you will get a call from a hospital that needs to send records to a specialist whose number you cannot remember. You will say "hold on" and find it in 30 seconds because you wrote it down. That is the goal.

4. Medical History

This is the one that nobody does, and the one that matters most when something goes wrong. You need a one-page summary of your loved one's medical history that you can hand to a new provider in 60 seconds.

Include:

- Diagnoses (with dates if you have them)
- Major surgeries (year, hospital, what was done)
- Allergies — and what reaction ("hives" vs "anaphylaxis" matter a lot)
- Implanted devices (pacemakers, stents, joint replacements)
- Recent hospitalizations
- Code status / advance directive (more on this later)
- Primary care provider's name and phone

Update it every six months or when major changes occur. Bring it to every new specialist. The amount of time and stress this saves is unreal.

The System That Actually Works (Pick One)

Here's where most people blow it — they buy a $40 binder with twelve color-coded tabs and never open it because it's too precious to mess up. Don't do that. Pick one of these three systems, whichever fits your brain, and start messy.

System A: The Binder (Old School, Reliable)

A 2-inch three-ring binder with these tabs:

- Insurance (cards, EOBs, denial letters)
- Medications (current list, plus old ones for reference)
- Contacts (the list above)
- Medical history (one-pager, plus past records)
- Appointments (calendar printouts, after-visit summaries)
- Bills (sorted by date)
- Notes (a legal pad for jotting things at appointments)

This system is bulletproof. The downside is that it's heavy and you have to physically carry it. The upside is that nothing is going to die or update itself or charge you a subscription.

System B: The Google Drive/One Drive/ Apple Cloud

Make one folder in an online cloud platform called "Medical." Inside it, save:

- Photos of insurance cards (front and back)
- A photo of the current medication list
- A photo of the medical history one-pager
- After-visit summaries (most patient portals let you download these as PDFs)
- Your loved one's date of birth and Social Security number — typed in a note that's locked behind your face ID

This is the system I use most days. It's always with me. It dies if my phone dies, which is why I also keep a paper backup at home. But I was also able to access it from any device with an internet connection.

System C: The Hybrid

Phone for daily access. Binder at home for the long haul. Honestly, this is what most people end up doing once they realize neither system alone is enough.

Sharing the Load (The Family Group Chat)

If there are other family members involved — parent, siblings, kids

— set up a group text or shared note where information lives. The rule: facts go in the chat, feelings can go anywhere else.

"Mom's potassium was 3.4 today, they're adding a supplement" goes in the chat. "I can't believe Aunt Linda hasn't visited" goes to your therapist.

I was fortunate and blessed with great in-laws. And I am not saying it just because they will probably read this book but because it is true. But I have seen it happen with other families and experienced it with other relatives. It sucks when someone is ill and others only want to fight. So, save yourself the hassle and keep to the facts.

This sounds harsh. It saves families.

Reducing Chaos Before It Starts

Caregiving is going to throw chaos at you no matter what. The goal is to reduce the chaos that comes from disorganization, so you have bandwidth left for the chaos you can't control.

A few moves that pay off forever:

- **Set up the patient portal.** Every major health system has one. It will let you message providers, view labs, request refills, and see appointments. It is not optional. Set it up the first week.
- **Sign a HIPAA release.** Without it, providers cannot legally talk to you about your loved one's care. Most offices have a one-page form. Sign one at every practice. Yes, every one.
- **Get a power of attorney for healthcare** if your person is willing and able. This is different from a financial POA. It lets you make medical decisions if they can't. You don't want to be figuring this out at 11 p.m. in an ICU.
- **Make one folder for bills, separate from EOBs.** I'll explain the difference later. For now, just don't mix them. They look similar. They're not.

Do This Next

- **Pick a system today.** Binder, phone folder, or hybrid. Don't agonize. Pick the one you'll actually use.
- **Start the medication list.** Type it, print two copies, fridge and bag. If you don't know all the doses, write what you know now. You'll fill in the rest.
- **Set up the patient portal** for your loved one's main provider. Sign in. Click around. Find the messages tab — that's the one you'll use most.
- **Sign a HIPAA release** at the next appointment, before the visit starts. Do not wait.
- **Pick one person** to share information with so you're not the sole holder of the entire family's medical knowledge.

Day one done. From here on, when anyone asks you what your loved one takes, when they were last seen, who their cardiologist is — you don't have to guess. You have a system. The system is ugly. The system is incomplete. The system works.

In the next chapter, we're going to talk about who all these people are. Because once you understand the players, the game gets a lot easier to play.

Chapter Three

Understanding the Healthcare Players

Who Does What, and Why That Matters

If you've ever sat in a hospital room and watched five people in scrubs walk through in 30 minutes, asked yourself who any of them are, and then nodded politely instead of asking — congratulations, you are a normal human in a healthcare setting.

Hospitals and clinics are full of people who all wear similar uniforms, use unfamiliar titles, and say things to your loved one that don't always get explained. The result is that families walk out of those rooms with half the information they needed and no idea who to ask for the other half.

Here is the cheat sheet I wish someone had handed me. We're going to walk through who each person is, what they actually do, what they don't do, and who you should call when you have a specific kind of problem.

Providers

In healthcare, "provider" is the umbrella term for anyone licensed to diagnose and treat. That includes physicians (MDs and DOs), Nurse Practitioners (NPs), and Physician Assistants (PAs). They have different training paths and different scopes of practice depending on the state, but in most clinical settings, all three can examine, diagnose, prescribe, and manage care.

When someone refers to "the provider," they could mean any of them. Here's how they break down by role:

Primary Care Provider (PCP)

This is the quarterback. Internal medicine, family medicine, or geriatrics — depending on age and need. The PCP knows your loved one's whole picture, manages chronic conditions (diabetes, blood pressure, cholesterol), does annual physicals, and writes referrals to specialists.

This is the provider you should have a real relationship with. If your person doesn't have a PCP they trust, that's a fix-this-soon problem.

Specialists

Cardiologists, oncologists, neurologists, nephrologists — these are the providers who focus on one organ system or condition. They go deep on their thing. They usually don't manage anything outside their lane. So your cardiologist is going to focus on the heart, not the depression, even if the depression is making the heart problem worse.

This is why you need a PCP. Specialists do the deep work; the PCP makes sure the deep work doesn't accidentally contradict itself.

Hospitalists

This one surprises a lot of people. When your loved one is admitted to the hospital, their PCP usually does **not** see them. A separate provider — the hospitalist — manages care in the building. The hospitalist may or may not communicate with the PCP afterward. (This is why discharge follow-up matters so much. We'll get there.)

Hospitalists rotate, often weekly. So you may see Dr. Patel on Monday and Dr. O'Brien on Friday. They are looking at the same chart. They may have different styles. That's normal.

Surgeons

Surgeons cut. They consult before and after surgery, but they are not generally managing the long-term care plan. After a surgery, your surgeon is interested in the incision, the drains, and the immediate recovery. The PCP and specialists handle everything else.

Residents and Fellows (in teaching hospitals)

If you're at a university hospital, you'll see providers-in-training. Residents have their degree already and are doing supervised training. Fellows have finished residency and are subspecializing. They are real providers. They are also being supervised. If you have a question and a resident answers, you can absolutely ask, "Can you check with the attending and let me know?" — that's normal and welcome.

Nurses (We Are Not All The Same)

"The nurse" is not one role. It's about eight.

- **Registered Nurse (RN)** — assesses, gives meds, coordinates care, watches for changes. The nurse at the bedside is your single best source of information about what's happening hour to hour.
- **Licensed Practical Nurse (LPN/LVN)** — works under an RN's supervision in many settings, often in long-term care, doctors' offices, and clinics.
- **Certified Nursing Assistant (CNA)** — bathing, vitals, transfers, helping with meals. CNAs are the people who often know your loved one best because they spend the most time with them. Treat them like gold.
- **Medical Assistant (MA)** — technically not a nurse, but in most ambulatory clinics they are the person you interact with most.

They room patients, take vitals, update medication lists, and input information into the chart before the provider walks in. They are not licensed to assess or treat, but the information they capture shapes everything that happens next. Be accurate with them. They are often the first line.

- **Charge Nurse** — the RN running the floor that shift. If you have a problem and the bedside nurse can't fix it, the charge nurse is the next call.
- **Nurse Practitioner (NP)** — has additional training and can prescribe, diagnose, and manage care. In many practices, you'll see an NP more often than a doctor. That is not a downgrade. NPs are excellent.
- **Case Manager / Care Coordinator** — usually an RN or social worker. We'll talk about them in a minute. They are critical.

If you only remember one thing: the bedside RN is your most accessible expert. Use them. Be polite. Ask questions when they have a free hand.

Case Managers and Social Workers

These are the most underused humans in healthcare. They are also, very often, the ones who can solve the problems that everyone else hands you and walks away from.

A **case manager** (often an RN) coordinates the medical pieces — discharge planning, home health setup, durable medical equipment (walkers, beds, oxygen), insurance authorizations for services, transfers to rehab or skilled nursing facilities.

A **social worker** handles the human stuff — financial resources, transportation, food insecurity, mental health referrals, family conflicts, advance directives, and navigating Medicare/Medicaid applications.

A note on smaller hospitals: the case manager and social worker are often the same person. One human handling both the medical logistics and the human side of discharge. If you're not at a major medical center, don't go looking for two separate people — ask who handles discharge planning and work with whoever that is.

In my years working in ambulatory care, I had the privilege of watching case managers do their jobs up close. Those people can move mountains. They are the ones making sure that when your loved one leaves that hospital, they actually have what they need to leave safely. The home health referral is submitted. The hospital bed is delivered before the patient gets home. The oxygen is set up. The follow-up appointment is scheduled. None of that happens automatically. A good case manager is the reason it happens at all.

Ask for them by name within the first 24 hours of any admission. Get their direct number. They are the person who can actually move things — and unlike almost everyone else you'll encounter, moving things is literally their job.

Insurance (The Money Layer)

Insurance is its own ecosystem. We're going to spend the entire next chapter on it, but for now, just know there are usually three insurance-side people you might talk to:

- **Member services** — the number on the back of the card. They can answer benefits questions, eligibility, and explain coverage. Be patient with hold music.
- **Prior authorization team** — these are the people who decide whether a procedure or medication will be covered. You usually don't talk to them directly. The provider's office submits paperwork; this team approves or denies. If the insurance platform can't generate an automatic approval or denial, the request gets escalated to this team for manual review. That review takes time — and that delay is often where treatment gets held up.

- **Care management / case management at the insurer** — yes, the insurance company has case managers too. For complex conditions (cancer, transplant, complex chronic disease), they can sometimes unlock benefits and resources. Worth a call if your loved one's situation is complicated.

Important truth: insurance reps usually want to help. They are not the enemy — the system they're working inside of is. There's a difference, and keeping that straight will keep you from burning energy on the wrong fight.

On the facility side, most practices have their own prior authorization team as well. These are the staff who pull information from your loved one's chart and submit it to the insurance portal. Here's what most people don't know: these individuals are often not clinically trained. Many are high school graduates who have learned on the job. They are transcribing information from a chart into an online form. They are doing their best. They are also human — and as we saw in Chapter 1, a single transposed code can look like a denial that isn't one. This is not an indictment of those workers. It's a reason to verify.

Facilities

"Facility" is a word healthcare uses to mean any place that delivers care. It matters because where care is delivered changes how it's billed, who's in charge, and what happens next.

- **Hospital (acute care)** — for emergencies, surgeries, and complex illness. Highest cost. Highest intensity. Usually short stays.
- **Skilled Nursing Facility (SNF, pronounced "sniff")** — for short-term rehab after a hospital stay (PT, OT, IV antibiotics, wound care). Medicare covers a limited number of days under specific conditions.
- **Long-term care / nursing home** — for ongoing custodial care. Mostly not covered by Medicare; this is where Medicaid and

private pay come in.

- **Assisted Living** — housing with help (meals, meds, bathing). Mostly private pay.
- **Home Health** — nurses, aides, and therapists who come to the house for short-term skilled care. Covered by Medicare under specific rules.
- **Hospice** — comfort-focused care at the end of life. Can happen at home, in a facility, or sometimes in a hospice house. Covered by Medicare.
- **Outpatient clinics** — same-day visits, no overnight.

These categories matter because they have completely different billing structures, coverage rules, and discharge logic. “Skilled” vs “custodial” is a single word that will determine whether Medicare pays $15,000 or $0.

Who to Call and When (Quick Reference)

Save these mental rules. They will save you hours.

- **Question about a medication** → call the pharmacy or the prescribing provider. Pharmacists are wildly underused. They are drug experts.
- **New symptom that isn’t an emergency** → call the PCP’s office during business hours.
- **Trouble getting a procedure scheduled or authorized** → call the provider’s office first, not insurance. The provider has to submit the paperwork. Insurance often can’t do anything until they receive it.
- **Question about a bill** → call the billing department on the bill, not the provider.
- **Question about what insurance will cover** → call member services (number on the back of the card).
- **Question about a hospital admission, discharge plan, or**

rehab placement → ask for the case manager.

- **Concern about something happening on a hospital floor right now** → bedside nurse, then charge nurse, then nursing supervisor. (We'll go deeper on this in Chapter 10.)
- **Mental health crisis** → 988 (Suicide & Crisis Lifeline) or 911.
- **Stroke, chest pain, severe difficulty breathing, sudden confusion** → 911. Do not drive.

How to Communicate Effectively

A few small habits will make every conversation in healthcare go better:

- **Identify yourself and your relationship up front.** "Hi, I'm Tiffany, I'm John Smith's daughter, his date of birth is 4/12/1948." That gets through the first 30 seconds of bureaucracy.
- **State the purpose of the call in one sentence.** "I'm calling because we got a denial letter for Mom's MRI and I need help figuring out what to do next."
- **Take the name of every person you talk to.** First name, role, date, time. Write it in your notebook. "Talked to Maria, member services, 3/12 at 2:14 p.m. Said the auth was approved on 3/10, ref #ABC123." This single habit will save you when stories don't match later.
- **Repeat back what you heard.** "So just to make sure I understand — you're saying the appeal has been received, and we should hear back within 30 days?"
- **Ask what happens next.** Always. "What's the next step? When should I expect to hear something? Who do I call if I haven't heard by then?"

Do This Next

- **On a single page in your notebook, write down the names and roles of everyone currently involved in your loved one's care.**

PCP, specialists, pharmacy, home health (if any), case manager (if any). Phone numbers next to each.

- **Identify the gap.** Is there a PCP? Is there a case manager? If not, those are your next two calls to make.
- **The next time you're on the phone with anyone in healthcare, write down their name and the time of the call.** Build the habit now.

Now you know who's who. Next chapter, we're going to talk about the player nobody understands — and the one that determines whether you can actually get the care you need.

Insurance. Take a breath. We're going in.

Chapter Four

Decoding Insurance (Without Going Insane)

The System Is Confusing on Purpose. Here's How to Read It.

If you've ever read an insurance document and thought, "This is written in a language that resembles English but isn't," you are correct. Insurance documents are written by lawyers for other lawyers, with the assumption that you will give up. Most people do.

You don't have to become an insurance expert. You just need to understand five things: the basic terms, the difference between a referral and a prior authorization, why things get denied, how long any of this realistically takes, and where to look on your specific policy when something comes up. We're going to walk through all five.

The Five Terms You Have to Know

1. **Premium**

The amount paid every month to have the insurance at all. This is the price of the gym membership, regardless of whether you go to the gym.

2. **Deductible**

The amount you pay out of pocket each year **before** insurance starts paying its share. If your deductible is $3,000, you pay the first $3,000 of covered medical bills. After that, insurance kicks in.

Important: not every dollar you spend counts toward your deductible. Generally, payments for covered services count. Things insurance won't pay for at all (cosmetic procedures, certain experimental treatments) usually don't.

Plain example: Mom has a $3,000 deductible. She gets a $4,500 bill for a procedure. She owes $3,000 to hit the deductible. Then insurance starts paying its percentage on the remaining $1,500. (How much insurance pays depends on coinsurance — next term.)

3. **Coinsurance**

Once the deductible is met, you and insurance split costs by a percentage. Common splits are 80/20 (insurance pays 80%, you pay 20%) or 70/30.

Plain example: Same procedure. Deductible is met. The remaining $1,500 is split 80/20. Insurance pays $1,200. You pay $300.

4. **Copay**

A flat fee you pay at the time of service for certain visits or prescriptions. "$30 copay for primary care visits" means you pay $30 when you walk in, regardless of what the visit cost. Copays are separate from coinsurance.

Some services are copay-based; some are deductible-and-coinsurance based. The summary of benefits will tell you which is which.

(More on where to find that in a minute.)

5. Out-of-Pocket Maximum

This is the most important number in your entire policy and almost nobody pays attention to it.

It's the absolute most you have to pay out of pocket in a year for covered services. Once you hit it — through deductibles, coinsurance, and copays combined — insurance pays 100% of covered services for the rest of the year. (Premiums don't count toward this number.)

Plain example: out-of-pocket max is $9,000. Once you've paid $9,000 in deductible + coinsurance + copays during the plan year, you're done. Anything else covered for the year is fully paid by insurance. This number is why people with chronic, expensive conditions sometimes hit the OOP max in February and then have a much cheaper rest of the year. It's also why timing — getting a procedure in November vs January — sometimes matters financially.

Authorizations vs Referrals (Not the Same Thing)

These two get confused constantly. They are different. Mixing them up will cost you weeks.

Referral

A referral is when your **PCP** sends you to a specialist. On many plans (especially HMOs), insurance won't pay for a specialist visit unless your PCP referred you to them. The referral is the PCP's office submitting a piece of paperwork (or a portal click) saying, "Yes, this person should see a cardiologist."

Where it goes wrong: families assume the referral is automatic. It isn't. Sometimes the PCP forgets, the staff misses it, or the referral expires. If you scheduled a specialist appointment and you have an HMO plan, **call both offices ahead of time** to confirm the referral is in place.

Prior Authorization (PA, also called "pre-auth" or just

"auth")

Prior authorization is when **insurance has to approve a specific service** before it happens. MRIs, CT scans, certain medications, surgeries, home health, durable medical equipment, and most non-emergency hospital admissions can require PAs.

The PA is submitted by the **provider's office**, not by you. They send insurance the diagnosis (in code form), the procedure they want to do (in code form), and clinical notes explaining why.

Insurance reviews. They approve, deny, or ask for more information.

How Long Does Any of This Take?

Set your expectations now and you will save yourself a lot of agony.

- **Standard prior authorization:** typically 5 to 14 business days. Sometimes faster, sometimes slower. Two weeks is normal, not a delay.
- **Expedited / urgent prior authorization:** 24 to 72 hours. The provider has to mark the request as urgent — meaning waiting would seriously jeopardize health.
- **Referrals:** usually faster — often same day to a few days, depending on the practice.
- **Appeals after a denial:** 30 to 60 days for a standard appeal. Faster for urgent.

Translation: if your loved one needs an MRI and the doctor orders it today, do not be surprised if the appointment isn't scheduled for two to three weeks. The scheduling delay is usually not the imaging center being booked. It's the auth not being back yet.

Why Insurance Denies Things

Here's something most people don't know: most denials are not because insurance is evil. They are because of paperwork.

The most common reasons for denial:

- **The PA wasn't submitted at all.** The provider's office forgot, was waiting on something, or assumed it wasn't needed. Surprisingly common.
- **The diagnosis code didn't justify the service.** Insurance has rules: an MRI of the lumbar spine has to be paired with a back-related diagnosis, with documentation that conservative treatment was tried first. If the chart didn't say that, the auth gets denied.
- **Missing clinical notes.** The provider sent the request but not the supporting documentation. Insurance asks for more info. The office is slow to send it. Things sit.
- **Out-of-network provider.** The doctor or facility isn't in your plan's network.
- **Service is excluded under the plan.** Some things — cosmetic procedures, certain experimental treatments, some forms of long-term care — are simply not covered.
- **The clock ran out.** Many auths must be requested within a certain window before the service. Miss it, and they say no.

Knowing this changes everything. Most denials are fixable. We will go deep on appeals in Chapter 13. For now, just know: a denial is not a final answer. It is the start of a conversation.

A few days before my husband's Gamma Knife procedure, we got the call again. Insurance hadn't authorized it. Treatment might not happen.

I was sitting in a Walmart parking lot. I'd just done a grocery pickup after getting off work. I called the insurance company from my car and I stayed on that phone for over an hour.

The rep couldn't find a prior authorization request anywhere in the system. Not pending. Not denied. Not approved. He dug and dug, and finally found what appeared to be the problem: the request looked as though it had never been placed at all. It was sitting in the provider portal, incomplete — waiting for someone to attach the clinical notes supporting the need for Gamma Knife and hit send. Nobody had. It had just been sitting there.

By the time we figured that out, it was 5:03 p.m.

I tried to reach the CEO and president of the health system responsible because I was pissed and someone needed to be held accountable. One person holds both titles. I am not someone who bluffs about that kind of thing. I was not bluffing. Nobody put me through, because it was three minutes past the end of their business day.

I want to be clear about what was at stake: my husband had a brain tumor. He had a procedure scheduled. And the only reason it was in jeopardy was because someone hadn't hit submit.

The next day, calmer, I recognized that the man holding both titles had bigger problems on his desk than mine. But that didn't mean nothing happened. There's a process for situations like this — a way to make sure the right people know what went wrong without it becoming a screaming match that goes nowhere. I'll tell you how to use it in Chapter 9.

That's the thing about denials — and non-submissions, which are somehow even more maddening. They rarely mean no. They mean something is incomplete. A missing attachment. A form sitting in a queue. A box that didn't get checked. The fix is almost always findable. But you have to be the one who goes looking, because no one is going to call you to say they forgot.

His procedure went forward. I made sure of it.

Special Cases You Should Know About

Medicare

If your loved one is over 65, they're probably on Medicare. The basics:

- **Part A** — hospital insurance. Mostly free for people who paid into Medicare during their working years.

- **Part B** — outpatient and provider visits. Has a monthly premium and an annual deductible.
- **Part C (Medicare Advantage)** — private plans that bundle A, B, and usually D. Often have lower premiums but more rules and narrower networks.
- **Part D** — prescription drug coverage.
- **Medigap** — supplemental insurance to fill the gaps in Original Medicare.

Medicare Advantage is where families often get burned. The plans look great until something complex happens, and then the prior authorizations and network restrictions hit hard. Original Medicare + a Medigap plan tends to be more flexible, but more expensive month to month.

Medicaid

State-run, income-based, covers people with limited resources. Rules vary wildly state to state. If your loved one has a long-term care situation and is running through their savings, talk to a social worker or elder-law attorney about Medicaid planning before you're broke. The five-year lookback rule is real and brutal.

Dual Eligible (Medicare + Medicaid)

Some people qualify for both. The interaction is complicated and the benefits are real. Ask a social worker or a State Health Insurance Assistance Program (SHIP) counselor — they exist in every state, are free, and they actually know this stuff.

Worksheet: Know Your Insurance

That last piece — knowing where to look in your specific policy — is what this worksheet is for. Sit down with your loved one's insurance card and their summary of benefits (most insurers post it on the member website, or you can call and request it). Fill in the answers below for each plan you're dealing with. This single sheet will save you hours later.

Insurance company name: __________

Plan name: __________

Plan type (HMO, PPO, EPO, Medicare Advantage, etc.) : __________

Member ID: __________

Group number: __________

Customer service phone (back of card): __________

Annual deductible (in-network): $__________

Annual out-of-pocket maximum (in-network): $__________

Coinsurance percentage (in-network): __________

PCP copay: $__________

Specialist copay: $__________

ER copay: $__________

Urgent care copay: $__________

Does this plan require referrals? Yes / No

Where do I check authorization status? (portal URL or phone): __________

Plan year (calendar year, or some other 12-month period?): __________

Do This Next

- **Fill out the Know Your Insurance worksheet** above. You don't have to know it by heart, you just need to be able to find the answers in 30 seconds when someone asks you.
- **Create an online account** at the insurance company's member portal. Most denials and EOBs show up there before they show up in the mail.
- **Find out the renewal date** of the plan year. Plans often reset on January 1, but not all of them — Medicare Advantage plans run

on the calendar year, but employer plans sometimes run July to June. This matters for deductibles and OOP maxes.

- **Make a single rule for yourself:** every time you get a letter from insurance, you will not throw it away, even if it looks like junk. Especially if it looks like junk. Half the EOBs I see in the wild were nearly tossed.

That's the foundation. You now know more about insurance than most people, including most patients. We're not done with insurance — we'll come back to denials and appeals later — but the next chapters are about navigating actual care: appointments, referrals, urgent vs ER, and hospital stays.

Get a snack. Take a walk. Then meet me in Chapter 5.

Chapter Five

What's Actually Happening in That 15-Minute Appointment

Why Visits Feel Rushed (Because They Are)

You blocked off your morning. You drove your mom across town. You waited 40 minutes in the lobby. You finally got into a room. The medical assistant took vitals, asked some questions, then disappeared. You waited another 15 minutes. The doctor walked in, looked at the chart, asked three questions, told you the plan, said "any questions?" — and was out the door before you could remember the four things you wanted to ask.

If that has ever happened to you, I want you to know: it is not because the doctor doesn't care. It is because the appointment was scheduled for 15 minutes and the doctor has six more patients waiting, all of whom drove across town and waited 40 minutes. The system is squeezing everyone.

Once you understand the machine, you can work with it instead of getting flattened by it.

What the Provider Is Juggling Behind the Scenes

Most primary care visits are scheduled in 15- to 20-minute slots. Specialists may have 30 minutes for a new patient, 15 for follow-ups. In that time, the provider has to:

- Review the chart (if they have time before the visit)
- Read the MA's notes about what you said today
- Listen to your concerns
- Examine your loved one
- Make decisions about diagnosis and treatment
- Order labs, imaging, or referrals
- Document everything in the chart (this often takes longer than the visit itself)
- Submit billing codes
- Send messages, refill requests, and prior authorization paperwork

They are also being measured on quality metrics, satisfaction scores, and how well they're meeting documentation requirements. Many of them are doing notes on their lunch break and answering portal messages at 10 p.m. They didn't pick this pace. The system did.

None of that is your problem to solve. But it explains why you have to be ready — because they don't have time to draw the information out of you.

How Decisions Actually Get Made

Doctors don't decide one thing at a time. They walk into a room with a few likely diagnoses already in mind based on the chart, and they're asking questions to confirm or rule out each one. They are also doing math in their head about probability — how likely is each possibility, given age, history, and what they're seeing right now.

This is why **how you describe a symptom matters more than you think**. "She's been tired" gets one mental file. "She fell asleep in the middle of dinner three nights this week — that has never happened before" gets a completely different file.

Specifics. Specifics. Specifics. We'll come back to this.

How to Prepare BEFORE the Appointment

Most of the value of an appointment is created before you walk in. The 15 minutes in the room is the smallest part. Here is what to do in the days leading up:

Three Days Before

- **Confirm the appointment** — date, time, location, address. Look at the address. Look at it again. Specialists have multiple offices.
- **Confirm the referral and authorization** are in place if needed.
- **Pull together the records** — labs, imaging reports, hospital discharge papers from the past 6–12 months. Most patient portals will let you download these as PDFs. Print them or save them to your phone.

The Day Before

- **Make the symptom timeline.** When did it start? What does it feel like? What makes it better or worse? Has it changed? Is it constant or comes and goes?
- **Update the medication list** if anything has changed. (Though if you read Chapter 2 already, you know to keep this one updated.)
- **Write down your top 3 questions.** Not 12. Three. We'll talk about why.

The Morning Of

- **Bring the list of meds, the symptom timeline, the questions, your insurance card, and ID.**
- **Bring water and a snack** for your loved one if they may have to wait a while.
- **Plan to arrive 30 minutes early** — for parking, paperwork, and bathroom. You want to be in the line waiting to be registered 15 minutes before your appointment starts, not driving around the parking lot trying to find a spot.

The "Go In With This" Checklist

Print this and put it in your binder. Take it to every appointment.

- ☐ Photo ID and insurance card
- ☐ Updated medication list (printed)
- ☐ Symptom timeline / what's changed since last visit
- ☐ Top 3 questions written down
- ☐ List of other doctors involved + recent procedures or hospitalizations
- ☐ Pen and notebook (or phone with notes app open)
- ☐ Referral or authorization confirmation, if relevant
- ☐ Recent lab/imaging reports if seeing a new provider
- ☐ HIPAA release filed at this office (if it's your first visit as the caregiver)

The Top 3 Questions Rule

Here is the hard truth about appointments: you can't get every question answered in 15 minutes. If you walk in with a list of 12, the doctor will pick the three they think are most important and answer those, while you sit there feeling like you didn't get to your real concern.

Take the power back. Decide which 3 are most important to **you** before you walk in. Lead with them. Get those three answered, in order, before anything else.

Anything that doesn't get answered, write down. Send through the patient portal afterward. Or save it for the next visit. Or, if it's truly urgent, ask: "Can I schedule a follow-up in two weeks specifically for these other questions?"

I never had the experience of walking out of an appointment empty-handed because I'd brought too many questions. Not because I'm naturally organized, but because I'd spent enough time on the other side of the exam room door to know what happens when a family comes in with a legal pad full of items.

The provider does their best. They pick the two or three that seem most clinically urgent. The family leaves feeling like they ran out of time. Nobody's fault. Just math.

So I came in with two or three questions. Every time. Not because I didn't have more — I always had more — but because I knew which ones required a face-to-face answer and which ones could wait. Anything that needed a real conversation, I prioritized and brought with me. Anything else, I sent through the portal as it came up — and usually had an answer within hours to a few days.

It meant I almost always walked out having gotten what I came for. It also meant his providers trusted that when I reached out, it was for a real reason — not a list of twelve things I'd been saving up. That trust matters. Over time, the providers who knew me knew that if I was concerned, it was worth taking seriously. You build that by being precise, not by being loud.

Questions You Should Always Ask

Regardless of what the visit is about, these questions almost always pay off:

- **"What is the diagnosis, in plain English?"** If they say "essential hypertension," you say "so, high blood pressure with no specific cause we found?" Translate. Repeat back. Confirm.

- **"What are we doing about it, and why this approach over others?"** This invites the doctor to share their thinking. You learn a lot.
- **"What should we watch for that would mean we need to call sooner?"** This single question has caught more bad outcomes than I can count.
- **"What's the next step, and when should I expect it?"** Lab? Imaging? Referral? Follow-up appointment? When?
- **"Is there anything I should be doing differently at home?"** Diet, exercise, medication timing, fall precautions, etc.
- **"How do I get ahold of you if I have questions between now and the next visit?"** Portal? Nurse line? After-hours? Know before you leave.

How to Walk Out With What You Actually Need

Three small habits. They make a giant difference.

- **Take notes during the visit.** Phone, paper, doesn't matter. "Cardiologist: heart looks stable, holding meds same. Add lasix only if swelling gets worse. Recheck labs in 6 weeks." If your loved one is the patient, ask if they mind you writing things down. Almost no one minds.
- **Repeat the plan back before you leave.** "Just to make sure I have it right: we're starting metformin 500 mg twice a day, getting labs in 8 weeks, and following up here in 3 months. Did I get that right?" If anything is wrong, you find out now, not in the parking lot.
- **Get the after-visit summary.** Most clinics print one. If they don't print it, ask. It will list the diagnosis, plan, medication changes, and follow-up. Read it before you leave the building. If something's missing or wrong, fix it now.

Red Flags That Something Was Missed

Most appointments go fine. But sometimes you walk out with that prickly feeling that something didn't get addressed. Trust that feeling. Here are the most common things that get missed in rushed visits:

- **A new symptom didn't make it into the chart.** You said it. The MA didn't write it down. The doctor never saw it. Solution: ask, before leaving, "Can you confirm that the new chest pain symptom got documented and addressed today?"
- **A medication interaction wasn't checked.** New prescription was added. Old ones weren't reviewed. Ask: "Did we check this against the rest of her meds?"
- **A test result wasn't discussed.** You know something was drawn last visit and you never heard about it. Ask: "What did the labs from January show?"
- **Symptoms were attributed to something general ("it's just aging") without further workup.** Aging is real. So is missed pathology. If something feels new, ask: "Is there anything specific that could be causing this that we should rule out?"
- **The follow-up isn't scheduled.** "Come back in 3 months" is not the same as having an actual appointment on the calendar. Schedule before you leave.
- **The discharge instructions don't match what was said.** They tell you one thing in the room and the printed page says something else. Ask which is correct.

If You Are the Adult Child of an Older Parent

A specific note for this very common situation: doctors often default to talking to the patient, even when the patient is hard of hearing, mildly cognitively impaired, or simply soft-spoken. This is appropriate — your parent is the patient — but it can mean important details get lost.

Before the visit, ask your parent: "Is it okay if I jump in if I think we're missing something?" Most are relieved. Then in the room, sit where the provider can see you, take notes, and gently add information when needed: “Mom, you also mentioned the dizziness when you stood up — should we tell Dr. Chen about that?”

That phrasing — bringing the question back to your parent first — keeps the dynamic respectful while making sure the information actually gets there.

Do This Next

- **Print the “Go In With This” checklist** and put it in your binder or on the fridge.
- **For the next appointment, write your top 3 questions** on a sticky note and stick it to the front of the appointment paperwork.
- **Practice the repeat-back habit** at the next visit. Before you leave the room, say the plan out loud.
- **Set up the patient portal** if you haven’t already. Most follow-up communication and lab results live there.

Fifteen minutes is enough — if you know how to use it. You drove across town for this appointment. Walk out with something.

Next chapter: what to do when an appointment turns into a referral, and the referral turns into a waiting game. (Hint: don’t just wait.)

Chapter Six

Referrals, Authorizations, and Delays (The Waiting Game)

Why Things Sit. Why That's Normal. What to Do About It.

Your loved one's doctor said, "You need an MRI." That was Tuesday. It is now eight days later. The imaging center hasn't called. The doctor's office is suddenly hard to reach. You're refreshing the patient portal like it's a slot machine. Your blood pressure is climbing.

Welcome to the waiting game. It is universal. It is exhausting. It is also navigable, once you know what's actually happening behind the scenes.

In this chapter we're going to make the invisible visible: what is a referral vs prior authorization, who submits what, where things get stuck, and exactly how to follow up without losing your mind or your relationship with the office staff.

Referral vs Prior Authorization (One More Time, Slowly)

Quick recap from Chapter 4, with more detail. These two words are not interchangeable, even though people use them that way.

Referral

A referral is your **PCP saying yes, see a specialist**. It's PCP-to-specialist. On HMO and many Medicare Advantage plans, insurance won't pay the specialist unless this is in place.

A referral does **not** approve a specific service. It approves the visit.

Prior Authorization

A prior authorization — from here on we'll call it a PA, because that's what everyone in healthcare calls it — is **insurance saying yes, you can have this specific service**. It applies to expensive things — MRIs, CTs, surgeries, certain medications, home health, durable medical equipment, hospital admissions for non-emergency procedures.

A PA is service-specific. "Approval to have a knee MRI on the right knee" doesn't carry over to "a brain MRI two months later." Each service is its own auth.

What Actually Gets Submitted

If you've ever wondered why this all takes so long, here's the inside view. When a provider's office submits a prior authorization, they have to send:

- **Patient demographics** — name, DOB, insurance ID, address.
- **The CPT code** — a 5-digit number for the procedure or service. Each procedure has its own code. "MRI of brain without contrast" has a code. "MRI of brain with contrast" has a different one. Get it wrong, get a denial.

- **The ICD-10 code** — the diagnosis code. There are tens of thousands of these. The one chosen has to justify why the procedure is needed. And it has to be truthful and accurate. If it isn't, this is fraud.
- **Clinical notes** — the office visit note, prior treatments tried, any relevant labs or imaging.
- **Sometimes: a letter of medical necessity** — a written argument for why the service is required.

All of this goes through a portal, fax, or phone call — but mostly anymore it is a portal. Then it goes to a reviewer at the insurance company — sometimes a clinical reviewer, sometimes an algorithm first. They check the codes against insurance criteria. They approve, deny, or pend ("send us more info").

The biggest delay is not the insurance company being slow. It's usually waiting for someone in the doctor's office to send the paperwork. This is one of the few things in healthcare you can actually speed up — by following up with the right person.

Why Things Stall or Get Denied

Most stalls fall into a few buckets:

- **The order was placed but never sent for auth.** The doctor entered "order MRI" in the chart, but the auth team didn't pick it up yet. Or the provider forgot to let the team know that one was ordered. Common in busy practices.
- **The wrong codes were used.** A diagnosis code that doesn't justify the procedure under insurance rules. (At this point, portals are not smart enough to flag whether the code entered is even valid — which is exactly what happened with my husband's authorization for Keytruda. The wrong code type was entered and the system just accepted it.)
- **Insurance is asking for more info.** A "step therapy" requirement (try cheaper option first), or documentation that conservative

treatment was tried.

- **The insurer's portal lost the request.** Yes, this happens. Faxes don't transmit. Portals time out. Things vanish.
- **Wrong insurance on file.** Someone changed plans, the office didn't update, the auth went to the old insurer.
- **Out-of-network.** The imaging center the office uses isn't in your plan.

None of these are the end of the world. All of them are fixable. The fix usually starts with one phone call to the right place, which we'll get to next.

Timeline Expectations

We covered timelines in Chapter 4, but the short version: standard auth is 5–14 business days, urgent is 24–72 hours. Add another 1–2 weeks for the service to actually get scheduled after approval. From order to appointment, two to four weeks is normal.

Set your expectations now and you'll spend a lot less time oscillating between hopeful and furious.

If your loved one's situation is genuinely time-sensitive, say so. Out loud. To the right person. The system has gears that can move faster, but only if someone's pushing them.

Who to Call First (Hint: Not Always Insurance)

This is the part that saves you the most time. The instinct, when something is stuck, is to call insurance. That is usually the wrong first call.

Step 1: Call the Provider's Office

Ask for the prior authorization team, the referral coordinator, or the medical assistant who works with your doctor. Use this script:

"Hi, I'm Tiffany, calling for John Smith, DOB 4/12/1948. Dr. Chen ordered an MRI of the brain on March 5th. I'm calling to check the status of the prior authorization. Has it been submitted, and do we have

an authorization number yet?"

Possible answers:

- **"It was submitted on the 6th, we're waiting on insurance."** → You now know it's actually with insurance. Time to call them.
- **"It's still in our queue, we'll get to it."** → Politely ask: "Is there any way to expedite this? It's been a week and Mom is in pain."
- **"I don't see anything in our system."** → The order didn't make it to the auth team. Ask the office to check directly with the doctor.
- **"We got a denial, we're working on it."** → Ask why, and what they need from you.

Step 2: Call Insurance (If Office Says It's With Them)

Now you call the number on the back of the card.

"Hi, I'm calling about a prior authorization for John Smith, DOB 4/12/1948, member ID 123456. Dr. Chen submitted on March 6th for an MRI of the brain. Can you tell me the status?"

Insurance will tell you: pending review, approved, denied, or pending more info. If it's pending more info, ask **what** info is missing and **who** they sent the request to. Then call the provider's office and tell them. Be the messenger.

Step 3: Document Everything

Every call: name of person you spoke with, date, time, reference number, what they said. Without this, you will get told contradictory things by different people and have nothing to go back to.

The "Kind But Persistent" Phone Strategy

Office staff are not the enemy. They are also overwhelmed, underpaid, and dealing with a hundred families who all think their case is the most urgent. The families who get things moved are not the loud ones. They are the calm, organized ones who call back at exactly the right intervals.

The rhythm:

- **Day 5–7:** First check-in call. "Just checking on the status of the auth submitted on the 6th."
- **Day 10–12:** If still nothing, second call. "I'm following up again. We're at almost two weeks and I want to make sure nothing fell through."
- **Day 14+:** Time to escalate. Ask to speak to the office manager or the specific PA staff member by name. Reasonable, calm, persistent.
- **If genuinely urgent:** Mention the symptoms or risk. "I'm worried because Mom's headaches have gotten significantly worse this week."

Always end with: "What's the next step, when should I check back, and is there anyone else I should be talking to?"

When my husband first started having vision problems, the ophthalmologist found no structural reason for what he was experiencing. Dave being Dave, he took that as "I'm fine" and tried to move on. The vision didn't move on.

It kept happening. Same issue, same frequency, no explanation. That's when I pushed. I asked his PCP for a referral to a second ophthalmologist and requested a CT — head, chest, abdomen — because something was wrong and we didn't have an answer yet. Not a structural eye problem. Something else.

His PCP could have said no. The first ophthalmologist had already cleared him. On paper, there was nothing left to look for. But I knew my husband, and I knew that vision doesn't just do that for no reason.

That CT is what found the recurrence. Stage three renal cell cancer, back in his pancreas and liver — and we caught it early enough to fight it. I believe with everything I have that the two years we had after that diagnosis were made possible by not accepting the first answer.

Persistence isn't just about phone calls and authorization numbers. Sometimes it's about trusting what you know about your person and refusing to let the system tell you there's nothing to see.

If a PA Gets Denied

Don't panic. Most denials are not final. We'll go deep on appeals in Chapter 13. For now, here's the immediate move:

- **Read the denial letter.** Find the reason.
- **Call the provider's office.** Tell them. They often will resubmit with more documentation, called a "peer-to-peer" review where the ordering doctor talks to a doctor at the insurance company. Many denials get reversed at this step.
- **Ask for a copy of everything submitted.** Your right. Get the records.
- **If still denied, file a formal appeal.** (See Chapter 13.)

Special Situations

Step Therapy (a.k.a. Fail First)

Some plans require you to try a cheaper drug first and have it fail before they'll approve a more expensive one. This is infuriating when your doctor knows the cheaper one won't work, but it is a common rule. Ask your doctor about "step therapy override" if there's a clinical reason to skip the first drug.

Out-of-Network Exceptions

If the only specialist who can do something specific is out of network, sometimes insurance will cover them at in-network rates. This is called a **network gap exception** or **out-of-network authorization**. Ask both the provider and insurance about it. It is worth the call.

Urgent Authorizations

If something genuinely cannot wait — new cancer diagnosis, severe symptoms, post-discharge needs — the provider can mark a request as urgent. This shortens the timeline to 24–72 hours. If you think your situation qualifies, say so explicitly: "This feels urgent. Can it be submitted as expedited?"

Scripts You Can Steal

Calling the Provider's Office

"Hi, this is Tiffany calling for John Smith, DOB 4/12/1948. Dr. Chen ordered [procedure] on [date]. I'm calling to check on the prior authorization. Can you tell me whether it's been submitted, and if so, the status?"

Calling Insurance Member Services

"Hi, I'm calling on behalf of John Smith, member ID 123456, DOB 4/12/1948. There's a prior authorization request from Dr. Chen's office for [procedure], submitted on [date]. Can you tell me the status, and if there's any missing information?"

When You Get Stonewalled

"I understand. Can you tell me who I should be talking to next, and what the supervisor's name is in case I need to escalate?"

Do This Next

- **Add a column to your appointment calendar called "Auth status."** For every order placed, write the date and what's pending.
- **Set a reminder on your phone for day 5 after any auth was ordered.** That's your first check-in day.
- **Save these phrases in a note on your phone:** the scripts above. You'll use them more than you think.
- **Get the direct number for the prior auth team at your loved one's main practice.** Often this isn't on their website. Ask. Save it.

In the next chapter, we're going to talk about something simpler but no less important: when to use primary care, urgent care, or the ER. Get this wrong and you can waste hours, money, or a serious moment. Let's get it right.

Chapter Seven

Urgent Care vs Primary Care vs ER (Stop Guessing)

Where to Go, When, and Why It Actually Matters

Caregiving is full of 9 p.m. judgment calls. Mom's blood pressure is 180/95. Dad fell, got up, says he's fine, but his arm hurts. Your aunt has a fever of 102 and is confused. You're looking at the clock, the parking lot, and your phone, asking yourself the same question every caregiver eventually asks: ER, urgent care, or wait until morning?

Pick wrong and you'll either spend six hours and a thousand dollars in an ER for something a clinic could have handled, or you'll wait for an appointment while a real emergency unfolds. Both happen all the time. This chapter is going to give you a simple framework so you don't have to guess.

My Rule of Thumb

This is the rule I use, in plain English. Memorize it.

- **If you think they could die, or be permanently harmed, in the next few hours → ER.**
- **If it's annoying but not dangerous → urgent care or a walk-in clinic.**
- **If it's ongoing or routine → primary care.**

Three sentences. Most situations fit one of them. If you're standing in the kitchen at 11 p.m. and you don't know which one applies, default up. ER over urgent care, urgent care over waiting. Better safe than dead.

Primary Care: The Default Most People Skip

Primary care is the right answer for most things, most of the time. People skip it because they think the doctor is too busy, or because they don't want to be the patient who calls about "nothing."

Use primary care for:

- Ongoing or worsening chronic conditions (blood pressure trending up, diabetes harder to control, swelling getting worse)
- New symptoms that aren't dramatic but are persistent (fatigue, mild pain, sleep changes)
- Medication adjustments and refills
- Lab follow-up and screening
- Mental health symptoms (depression, anxiety, sleep issues)
- Routine illness (cough that's been around for a few days, sinus stuff that's not crushing)
- Anything you'd want a doctor to be aware of even if it doesn't feel urgent

Most PCP offices have same-day or next-day appointments for established patients. They don't always advertise this. Call and ask: "Mom is having [symptom]. Can she be seen today?" The answer is yes more often than you'd think. The trick is to call early in the morning.

If your PCP can't see you, they often have a triage nurse who can advise by phone. Ask. They'll tell you whether to go to urgent care, the ER, or wait.

Now here is a harsh truth: do not wait until 5 p.m. on a Friday and expect an answer. If your loved one is having issues earlier in the week, address them then. Not at 5 p.m. on a Friday. I wouldn't even wait until noon or 8 a.m. Friday. And that goes for Thursday if your PCP works just four days a week. The people who work in clinics are humans with families, just like you. They are looking forward to their weekend just like you do, and if they have the opportunity to leave a couple of hours early on the last day of their week, they sure as shit will. Just like you would. So don't procrastinate. If you do, that's on you, not them. Own that now that you've read this.

Urgent Care: The Middle Lane

Urgent care (or walk-in clinics, or "MinuteClinics") is for things that need attention today but aren't life-threatening. They handle the things primary care could handle, but on evenings, weekends, or when your PCP can't fit you in.

Use urgent care for:

- Mild to moderate fevers
- Common infections (UTIs, sinus, ear, sore throat)
- Minor lacerations needing stitches
- Sprains and minor injuries
- Mild allergic reactions (no breathing trouble)
- Skin issues (rashes, infections, not getting better on their own)
- Mild dehydration
- Routine prescription bridges if you're stuck

Important caveat for older or medically complex patients: urgent care is good at simple problems on otherwise healthy people. They are usually not equipped for complex elderly patients with multiple conditions. If your loved one has heart failure, kidney disease, or is on blood thinners, the threshold to go to the ER instead is lower. A "minor fall" on a blood thinner is not minor. A urinary tract infection in someone with dementia can crash them in hours. When in doubt, ER.

Also: not all urgent care is created equal. Some are true urgent cares and bill as such. Some are walk-in clinics and bill no differently than a visit to your PCP. Some have x-ray, some don't. Some can do IV fluids, some can't. Some are open until 10 p.m., some close at 7. Know which one you'd actually go to **before** you need it. Save it in your phone.

One more thing: check that your urgent care is actually in-network before you walk in. Some are owned by hospital systems and bill at ER rates regardless of what the sign outside says. That's a mistake that can turn a $250 bill into a $2,500 one.

The Emergency Department

The ER is for the things that could kill or permanently harm someone. It is also expensive, slow, exhausting, and sometimes traumatic. Use it when you need it. Don't avoid it when you do.

Go to the ER (or call 911 — different decision; we'll get there) for:

- **Chest pain or pressure,** especially with shortness of breath, sweating, nausea, or pain spreading to arm/jaw/back
- **Sudden severe headache** (worst of their life)
- **Sudden weakness, numbness, or trouble speaking** (stroke signs — see below)
- **Severe difficulty breathing**
- **Severe abdominal pain** that won't let up
- **Major bleeding that won't stop with pressure**

- **Loss of consciousness** or unable to wake up
- **Confusion that is new** or significantly worse than baseline
- **Suicidal thoughts with a plan, or active mental health crisis**
- **Severe injury** (head injury with vomiting, suspected fracture, deep cut)
- **Severe allergic reaction** (swelling of face/throat, trouble breathing)
- **Signs of sepsis** (fever, rapid breathing, confusion, very low blood pressure, especially in elderly)
- **Falls in someone on blood thinners,** even if they "seem fine"

Stroke Signs: Memorize FAST

- **F**ace drooping
- **A**rm weakness
- **S**peech difficulty
- **T**ime to call 911

Time matters more in stroke than almost any other condition. Every minute counts. If you're seeing FAST signs, call 911. Do not drive.

ER vs 911

Call 911 — don't drive yourself or your loved one — when:

- Chest pain, especially with other symptoms above
- Stroke signs
- Severe difficulty breathing
- Loss of consciousness
- Severe injury that you can't safely move them with
- Suspected overdose

Paramedics can start treatment in the ambulance and call ahead, which often gets faster care once you arrive. Driving someone with chest pain to the ER is dangerous — to them and to other drivers if something gets worse on the way.

Drive yourself when: the situation is urgent but stable, the person can walk to the car, and you're alert enough to drive safely.

Cost Differences and Consequences

Money matters here, even though we wish it didn't.

- **PCP visit:** $20–$50 copay typical, sometimes covered fully on Medicare with a Part B doctor's visit cost share.
- **Urgent care visit:** $50–$150 typical, plus separate charges for x-ray, labs, or procedures.
- **ER visit:** $300–$1,500+ in copays alone, plus deductible and coinsurance on the actual charges, which can run thousands. Even a simple ER visit can leave you with a $2,000 bill.

Important: **never let cost stop you from going to the ER for a real emergency.** The bill is fixable. A heart attack walked off is not.

But: knowing the financial difference helps you avoid the ER for things that don't need it. Lots of urgent care visits get sent to the ER unnecessarily because the patient walked into the wrong door first. The ER will not turn you away, even if the issue could have been handled elsewhere.

Real-Life Examples

Example 1: Mom's Foot Hurts

She tripped over a rug yesterday. She didn't fall. Her foot is sore. She can walk on it. Mild swelling. No bruising.

Where to go: primary care, or urgent care if PCP can't see her in a day or two. Not the ER.

Example 2: Dad Fell

He fell getting out of the shower. He hit his head. He's on a blood thinner. He says he feels fine.

Where to go: ER. Now. Falls on blood thinners are an automatic ER trip even without obvious symptoms because of the risk of slow brain bleeds.

Example 3: Aunt Has a UTI

She's had UTIs before. Burning, urgency, classic symptoms. She is otherwise healthy.

Where to go: primary care or urgent care. Either works.

Example 4: Grandma Has a UTI and Suddenly Seems Confused

Same UTI symptoms, but she's also acting differently. More forgetful. Slurring slightly. Sleeping more.

Where to go: ER. New confusion in an elderly person can be sepsis, stroke, or other serious cause. Get her seen now.

Example 5: Chest Pain

Mid-afternoon. Pressure in the chest, slight shortness of breath.

Where to go: ER, by 911. Even if it turns out to be nothing, this is one of the symptoms you absolutely do not wait on.

Example 6: Fever

It's 8 p.m. and your loved one has a fever of 101. You've given Tylenol and it comes down.

Where to go: PCP or walk-in clinic the next day. A fever that responds to Tylenol and isn't accompanied by confusion, difficulty breathing, or severe pain can wait for morning.

The morning after Dave's Gamma Knife procedure, something was off. He was struggling to put his pants on — not in a tired, just-woke-up way, but in a way that was wrong. Like he couldn't sequence it. One leg, then the other. He kept losing track.

I took our son to daycare and came home. Then I handed Dave a piece of paper and a pen and asked him to write his name.

He couldn't do it. He tried for five minutes. He was furious with me for asking. He still couldn't do it.

I made him go to the ER.

Not the hospital where he had the procedure the day before — our local ER. And that was the right call. I was able to ensure he got the CT scan that showed significant brain swelling causing what's called a midline shift — his brain was being pushed off center by the pressure. From there, they arranged ambulance transport to the facility equipped to treat him properly.

I want to be clear about the decision I made in that moment: I didn't know what was wrong. I knew something was wrong. I didn't wait for it to get more obvious. I didn't call the cancer center first and wait on hold. I went to the nearest ER and let them figure out the next step.

That is exactly what the ER is for. You don't need a diagnosis to go. You need a reason to be worried.

Before You Go

If time allows, in any care setting:

- Bring the medication list.
- Bring the insurance card and ID.
- Bring a list of allergies.
- Bring a one-line summary of medical history ("78yo, heart failure, on warfarin, diabetes, recent hospital stay 2/15").
- Bring a phone charger, a snack, water, glasses, hearing aids.
- Bring a pen and paper for notes.

If you don't have time — going for a real emergency — go. Bring the phone with the photos of the meds and insurance. The rest is figure-outable from the car.

After the Visit

Three things, every time, no matter where you went:

- **Get the discharge summary.** Read it before you leave.
- **Schedule the follow-up.** ER and urgent care visits often say "follow up with PCP." Make the appointment **before you forget.**

Even if that means calling your PCP's office from the ED and leaving a voicemail to make sure the follow-up gets scheduled.

- **Update your records.** Add the visit to your notebook or app. Update the medication list if anything changed.

Do This Next

- **Today, save in your phone:** the address and phone number of your PCP, your preferred urgent care (with hours), and your closest hospital ER.
- **Memorize FAST.** Say it out loud. Teach it to your loved one if they're capable. If they live alone, post it on the fridge.
- **Make the rule simple:** could die in the next few hours → ER. Annoying but not dangerous → urgent care or walk-in. Ongoing → primary care. Default up if unsure.
- **Find out** if your PCP has a triage nurse line and what hours it's open. That's the call to make first when you're not sure.

Next chapter: what happens when your loved one ends up admitted. Hospital stays are their own universe — and the most important thing you can learn about them is what to ask, every single day.

Chapter Eight

Hospital Stays — What No One Explains

The Inside View of an Admission

Hospitals are loud, fluorescent, and disorienting. Your loved one is wearing a thin gown that doesn't close in the back. People keep walking in and out. Different doctors say slightly different things. Someone is talking about discharge before you've even gotten a clear answer about why your person is here.

If this has happened to you, you are not imagining it. Hospital stays move fast, and the systems that run them are designed for efficiency, not for family understanding. The good news is that hospitals are actually pretty predictable, once someone explains how they work. This chapter does that. By the end, you'll know who's in charge, when decisions get made, how to ask the right questions every single day — and how to make sure discharge doesn't blindside you.

What Happens When Someone Is Admitted

From the time your loved one is told they're being admitted, here's what's going on behind the scenes:

- An admitting physician (usually a hospitalist) takes over their care. **This is almost certainly not their PCP. The PCP may not even be notified.** I remember when PCPs would do rounds and take care of their own patients when they were admitted — but in most places, those days are gone. Your PCP is busy back at the clinic managing their other 2,500+ patients. You are now in the care of a hospitalist, whose entire job is to make sure admitted patients get the right care, the right treatment, and get home as soon as it's appropriately safe to do so.
- They get a bed assignment. Whether they go to a regular medical floor, a step-down unit, or the ICU depends on how sick they are.
- Orders go in. Labs, imaging, medications, monitoring, diet, activity level.
- A nurse takes over their bedside care. This nurse changes every 12 hours (day shift / night shift).
- Specialists may be "consulted." Cardiology, infectious disease, neurology, etc. — depending on the issue.
- A case manager or care coordinator gets assigned. Often within 24 hours. They're already starting to think about discharge.

Here's the thing nobody tells families: the moment your person is admitted, the team is already planning to discharge them. The financial and bed-availability pressure to move people through is constant. But honestly? Early discharge planning is also in the best interest of your loved one. People don't heal in hospitals. They're loud, your rest is constantly interrupted, and the risk of picking up an infection goes up the longer you're there. Most people don't want to be there — and they shouldn't stay longer than they need to. The goal is to get home as quickly and as safely as possible. This isn't sinister; it's how hospitals work. But it means **you** need to start asking discharge questions early, not at the end.

Rounds, Consults, and Who Is Making Decisions

Rounds

"Rounds" is when the hospitalist (and sometimes residents, students, pharmacists, and case managers) come around to discuss the patient. This is where decisions get made. It usually happens in the morning, but the exact window depends on the team's caseload and their schedule that day.

To get a better idea of when to expect them, ask your loved one's nurse — they'll usually know the typical time. But plan to be there at least 30 minutes before that window opens and 30 minutes after, just in case. Rounds don't wait for family.

This is the most important moment of the day for understanding what's happening. If you're trying to talk to the doctor, this is when they'll be in the room. If you can be there during rounds — even by phone — do it.

Consults

If your loved one has, say, a heart issue and a kidney issue, the hospitalist will "consult" cardiology and nephrology — meaning, ask them to weigh in. The hospitalist remains the primary doctor, but the consultants make recommendations.

This is why you see different doctors. They're not random. Each one has a reason. Ask the bedside nurse: "Who's been consulting on this case?" to keep track.

Why You See Different Doctors

Hospitalists work in shifts — usually 7 days on, 7 days off. So if your mom is admitted on Monday, you may see Dr. Patel through the weekend, then Dr. O'Brien starting next Monday. They are not starting from scratch — there's a handoff and a chart — but they may have slightly different styles or opinions. This is normal. If something feels inconsistent, ask the new doctor: "Can you walk me through your understanding of where we are?"

What to Ask DAILY

If you do nothing else in this chapter, do this. Every day your loved one is in the hospital, you should be asking these questions of either the bedside nurse, the hospitalist during rounds, or the case manager:

- "What changed in the last 24 hours, for better or worse?"
- "What is the working diagnosis right now?" (It can change.)
- "What are we doing today and tomorrow — tests, medications, plans?"
- "What are the criteria for discharge?" ("We need her oxygen off, eating, walking, and her labs stable.") Knowing the goal helps you understand the timeline.
- "What is the estimated date of discharge?" Even if it's a guess, ask. Plans are easier when you know the target.
- "Where will she go after discharge — home, rehab, skilled nursing?"
- "What questions or concerns do I need to bring up with the team today?" (Ask the bedside nurse this. They'll often tell you the truth.)

Write the answers in your notebook. The next day, ask again. You'll start to see the trend, which is more useful than any single day's report.

Discharge Planning (And Why It Often Feels Rushed)

Discharge is where most things go wrong. Families get blindsided. Patients leave without the right meds, equipment, or follow-up. People bounce back to the ER within a week.

Why? Because discharge usually gets decided in the morning and executed in the afternoon, often with the family caught off guard. The doctor says "she can go home today" at 9 a.m. By 2 p.m. they're handing you discharge papers and asking when you can come pick her up.

Don't let this catch you. Start the discharge conversation early — ideally on day one or two — because I can tell you that the care team already is. It's a known rule in healthcare that discharge planning should begin at the time of admission. What happens though is that it all gets done behind the scenes, or families are talked to but don't really understand what's being said. Don't wait for them to bring it to you. Start asking about discharge the day your loved one is admitted and keep asking every single day.

Questions to Ask About Discharge — Early

- Where is she going? Home? Rehab? Skilled nursing facility? Acute rehab? These have very different requirements and timelines.
- Who is the case manager? Get the name and direct number.
- What does she need at home? Oxygen, walker, hospital bed, IV antibiotics, home health visits, wound care?
- Who is going to set up the home health or equipment? Hospital case manager, or you?
- What follow-up appointments are needed, and by when? PCP within a week? Specialist within two? Get specific.
- What medications is she going home with, and have any been changed?
- Are any of those medications new and likely to require prior auth at the pharmacy?
- What do I do if something goes wrong tonight or tomorrow?

Going to a Skilled Nursing Facility (SNF) After Discharge

If the hospital stay ends with your loved one going to a rehab facility or skilled nursing facility instead of straight home, there are a few things you need to know before you agree to anything.

A skilled nursing facility — you'll hear it called a SNF, or sometimes "sniff," which is just how people say the abbreviation out loud — is a facility that provides medical care and rehabilitation after a hospital stay. Here's what to know:

- **Medicare covers a limited number of days (up to 100),** but only if certain conditions are met — a 3-day inpatient hospital stay first, plus a need for skilled care daily. After day 20, there may be a copay. Don't assume you know what your plan covers. Call the insurance company directly and ask them to walk you through the details before your loved one is discharged. You don't want to be caught off guard by a bill you weren't expecting.
- **"Inpatient" vs "observation" status matters.** If your loved one was on "observation status" in the hospital — even if they slept there for three nights — Medicare may not count it as an inpatient stay, which means SNF coverage could be denied. Ask the case manager directly: "Is she inpatient or observation status?" Ask early. Push back if needed.
- **You usually have a few facility choices.** The case manager will give you a list. Tour them if you can — they are not all the same. Read recent reviews. Ask about staffing ratios. If you live in a rural area like I do, you may have to travel further than you'd like. It's not ideal, but it's the nature of the beast. Not every community has a five-star SNF in its backyard.
- **Therapy schedule matters.** Ask each facility how many days a week physical therapy (PT) and occupational therapy (OT) are offered, and how many minutes per day. PT focuses on strength, mobility, and getting your loved one moving safely again. OT focuses on the practical stuff — getting dressed, bathing, using the kitchen — the daily tasks they need to be able to do before they can go home.

How to Not Get Blindsided by Discharge

- Have a discharge conversation by day two. Even if it feels premature.
- Identify the case manager and exchange phone numbers. This is the human who is going to be the most useful to you in the discharge process.
- Don't agree to a discharge if you're not ready. If the proposed discharge date doesn't work — equipment isn't in, home isn't safe, you can't be there — say so. The hospital can sometimes delay a day, especially if there's a clinical reason.
- Use the appeal right. If you genuinely believe discharge is premature, you have the right to appeal. Most hospitals must give you a notice called the "Important Message from Medicare" (or similar for other insurers) that explains how. The appeal review typically happens within 24–72 hours and discharge is delayed during it.

How to Push Back If Something Feels Off

Sometimes the plan doesn't sit right. The new medication didn't get explained. A test result wasn't followed up on. Your loved one seems worse than the team is acknowledging. Trust that feeling — and use the chain.

A lot of caregivers hesitate to speak up because they don't want to be seen as difficult, or they worry it will somehow affect how their loved one is treated. I understand that fear. But here's what I know from being on the inside: asking questions and raising concerns doesn't make you a problem. It makes you a present, engaged family member — and most staff respect that.

Let me tell you what speaking up actually looks like.

A few days after my husband Dave started his targeted oral treatment for renal cell cancer, he called me complaining of chest pain. If you've read anything about this man, you know he didn't complain unless there was a real reason. A visit to our local ER confirmed he was having a massive heart attack. One month after finding out his cancer had returned, he had a heart attack.

He was transferred to the facility where he was also being treated for cancer, so his oncologist could be involved in his care. The day after admission he had a heart catheterization, and we were told he had a blockage in the artery cardiologists sometimes call the "widowmaker." But they hadn't treated it yet — cardiology wanted to talk to oncology first. It was a Saturday. Things move slower on weekends.

Sunday came. It had been 24 hours since the cath and we still had no plan, no update, no answer. We were on the oncology floor because of Dave's history, but cardiology was running his care — and the two teams apparently hadn't connected yet. Every time I asked the nurse what was happening, I got a version of "we're waiting for cardiology and oncology to talk."

At some point I picked up the admission booklet that had been sitting on the bedside table — mostly out of habit, honestly. I was always reading how other facilities did things, looking for ideas I could bring back to my own. I came across a section called "Code Help." I read it carefully. It explained that family members could initiate a Code Help when they felt their loved one's condition was deteriorating, or when something about their care just wasn't right.

Here we were. Forty-eight hours after admission. Twenty-four hours after a heart cath for a widowmaker blockage. No treatment. No plan. No conversation between the two teams responsible for keeping my husband alive.

My husband was mortified when I told him what I was about to do.

I turned on his call light and waited for his nurse — the same nurse I'd been asking for updates all morning. When she came in, I held up the booklet, kept my voice calm and curious, and told her I'd just read about Code Help and wanted her honest opinion on whether I should call one, given that cardiology and oncology didn't seem to be connecting. I read her the passage directly from the booklet. I wasn't mean. I wasn't accusatory. I was just a wife who had read the fine print.

She asked me to hold on before I did anything. She wanted to make a phone call first.

Within ten minutes, both oncology and cardiology were in the room. Together. Making a plan. Dave was scheduled for a second heart cath the next morning to have a stent placed.

After they left, Dave apologized for getting upset with me. He said he was glad I'd done it — but he'd been afraid they would take worse care of him if I pushed.

Here's what I told him, and what I want you to hear: hospitals are evaluated constantly — by the federal government, by insurance companies, by patient satisfaction surveys. And they know, just like I do, that the people who aren't happy are the ones who fill out those surveys. Speaking up doesn't put your loved one at risk. Staying silent when something is wrong does.

So use the chain. Every hospital has one.

- **Talk to the bedside nurse first.** Frame it as a question, not an accusation: "I'm a little concerned about how Mom seems today — she was clearer yesterday. Has the team noticed?"
- **If that doesn't resolve it, ask for the charge nurse.** "Can I talk to the charge nurse about my concerns? I'd like to make sure the team is aware."
- **Then ask for the hospitalist or attending physician directly.** "I'd like to speak with Dr. Patel before the end of his shift. Can you let him know?"
- **If it's still not resolved, ask for the patient advocate or patient relations.** Every hospital has one. They are paid to help

patients and families navigate exactly these situations.

- **Read your admission booklet.** I mean it. Programs vary by hospital — Code Help, Rapid Response, Condition H — but many facilities give families the ability to escalate directly when something feels wrong. You won't know what tools you have unless you read it.
- **For acute clinical concerns, ask the nurse about the rapid response team.** If something is going wrong fast, this is the escalation that brings a team to the bedside immediately.

Things You Have a Right to Ask For

Before your loved one leaves that building, make sure you have these things. Don't assume anyone will hand them to you automatically — because they won't always. And sometimes the discharge process moves so fast that you may not even realize what you have because you don't know what you're looking at. Make sure you have each of these items and that the discharge nurse has explained them so you actually understand. Ask questions when you don't. **The nurse is not going home with you.**

- A copy of the discharge summary before you leave.
- Written instructions in plain language for medications, follow-up, and warning signs.
- A medication reconciliation — confirmation that the home med list now matches what they want her on.
- A printed list of new prescriptions sent to the pharmacy.
- Information about who to call if something goes wrong overnight or over the weekend.
- A patient advocate if there's a concern that hasn't been addressed.

Hospital Survival Logistics for the Caregiver

Hospitals are not designed for the people who love the patient. Here's how to survive being there:

- **Bring a charger and a charging brick.** Outlets near hospital beds are scarce, and the ones that exist may not be anywhere near where you're sitting. Get a cord with enough length to reach across the room.
- **Bring a sweater.** Hospitals can be cold, and you will be there longer than you think.
- **Eat.** There is a cafeteria. It is fine. Vending machines are also fine. And with modern conveniences, many hospitals now allow delivery services like DoorDash to drop off at the main lobby. When Dave was in the hospital, DoorDash was a lifesaver — sometimes you just need comfort food or something that doesn't taste like a cafeteria. Don't run yourself into the ground trying to be a martyr about meals.
- **Bring something to occupy your mind.** A laptop, tablet, book, or e-reader. When Dave was admitted for five days at a time during his CNS lymphoma treatment, I was able to work from my laptop right next to his bed. It kept me sane. Having some sense of normalcy in an abnormal situation matters more than you'd think.
- **Sleep at home if you can.** Hospital chairs will destroy your back and your judgment. The patient is being watched by professionals all night. You are allowed to rest. If the hospital is too far to drive back and forth daily — Dave's was an hour and a half from our home — ask the patient services office if there are nearby hotels that offer discounts for families of admitted patients. Most do. It costs more upfront but saves you from physical and mental breakdown later.
- **Figure out parking on day one.** Some hospitals have free parking. Others will charge you by the day and it adds up fast. Ask at the front desk or patient services office whether there's a reduced rate for families of admitted patients. Don't assume — just ask.
- **Take notes. Always.** Phone or paper. Names, times, plans.
- **Trade off with another family member if possible.** Care-

giving alone in a hospital is brutal. If you have someone who can step in and give you a break, use them. And I say that knowing how hard it is to actually do. I didn't let anyone help me at first — I was going to be there, period. That was just who I was. But somewhere around Dave's fourth or fifth admission I started to find a rhythm. I'd stay the first two nights, then go home, and come back to pick him up at discharge. It was a decision Dave and I made together. He was so well cared for at that point that we both agreed the one who needed me more was our three-year-old son at home. The grammies were doing a wonderful job — don't get me wrong. But nothing really replaces a momma when you're only three years old.

Do This Next

- **If your loved one is in the hospital right now,** ask the bedside nurse for the case manager's name and direct number. Today. Don't wait.
- **Set a phone reminder for daily 8:30 a.m. check-in** while they're admitted. That's your cue to ask the daily questions.
- **Find out what time rounding is, be there, and participate.** This is not the time to sit quietly in the corner.
- **Print the daily questions list and tape it inside your notebook now** — before you need it. Most hospital admissions aren't planned. You won't have time to find it later.
- **Read the admission booklet.** All of it. The tools available to you are only useful if you know they exist.
- **Memorize the chain of command:** bedside nurse → charge nurse → hospitalist → patient advocate. For acute concerns, ask about the rapid response team.

That's Part 2. You now know how the system actually works. Now it's time to make it work for you. Let's talk about advocacy.

Chapter Nine

How to Advocate Without Being "That Person"

Speaking Up Without Burning Down the Room

Let's talk about the caregiver who scares the nursing staff. You've seen that person. You've probably been terrified of becoming that person. This chapter is about why that fear, while understandable, might be getting in your way.

There's a fear most caregivers carry — that if they push too hard, ask too many questions, or call too often, they'll be labeled difficult. That somehow the staff will retaliate by giving worse care, or rolling their eyes, or treating their loved one like a number.

Here's the truth, from someone who's been on both sides: healthcare workers don't punish patients for engaged families. What they do, sometimes, is shut down around families who feel hostile, scattered, or impossible to satisfy. The difference between an advocate the team works with and a family the team avoids is **how**, not how much.

This chapter is going to teach you how to speak up in a way that gets results, without becoming the person staff dread seeing on the schedule.

Why You HAVE to Speak Up

Let's start with the non-negotiable: you have to speak up. Not sometimes. Always. Every appointment, every hospital stay, every phone call. Because if you don't, things get missed.

Healthcare is built on quick decisions, short visits, frequent hand-offs, and overworked staff. Every step is an opportunity for something important to fall through. The patients with the best outcomes are not the lucky ones. They are the ones whose families speak up — politely, persistently, specifically — at every step.

Your job as a caregiver is not to be agreeable. It's to be the second set of eyes the system needs, and often doesn't have.

How to Be Assertive but Effective

Effective advocacy has three ingredients:

- **Clarity.** Know what you're asking for, and what answer would satisfy you.
- **Calm.** Yelling, crying, or being sarcastic shifts the conversation from your concern to your behavior.
- **Specificity.** "This isn't right" gets ignored. "Mom's blood sugar has been over 300 for three days, and her insulin order hasn't changed — can we look at that?" gets results.

If you can do those three things, even imperfectly, you will be in the top 10% of advocates the staff will encounter today. I mean that.

What Actually Gets Results vs What Gets Ignored

What Gets Results

- **Asking specific clinical questions** with a clear ask: "Can we get a urinalysis to rule out a UTI?"
- **Naming what you observed** with concrete detail: "Yesterday

she was alert. Today she didn't recognize me."

- **Following the chain of command** when the first conversation doesn't resolve it.
- **Documenting and following up:** "I called yesterday at 2 p.m. and spoke with Maria; she said the order was put in. I'm following up because we still haven't received it."
- **Saying thank you when something goes well.** Yes, this matters. Staff who feel acknowledged are more responsive when issues come up.

What Gets Ignored (or Worse)

- **Vague venting:** "This place is a disaster."
- **Personal attacks on staff:** "You're terrible at your job." Even if you're frustrated. Especially if you're frustrated.
- **Threats:** "I'm going to sue you." Once that's said, the conversation usually ends and lawyers get involved. That's almost never what you actually want.
- **Constant calling about minor things.** I understand why it happens — you're scared and you want answers. But when everything is urgent, nothing is. Save your fire for the moments that matter.
- **Refusing to listen.** Advocacy is a two-way conversation. If you've already decided the team is wrong before they've explained, you'll miss information you need.

The Scripts That Work

If you're not used to speaking up, the first few times feel awkward. And in a stressful medical moment, your brain will go blank at exactly the wrong time. That's why having specific words ready matters. These phrases are short, calm, and get the conversation moving. Steal them.

When You Don't Understand

"I need clarification on what you just said. Can you explain it again

— maybe in plainer language?"

This is one of the most powerful things you can say. It costs nothing, and it almost always gets you a clearer answer. Don't be embarrassed. Most people in the room don't understand either.

When You Want to Understand the Reasoning

"Can you walk me through why we're choosing this approach over another option?"

This invites the doctor to share their thinking instead of just telling you the conclusion. It also gently signals that you want to be a participant, not just a passenger.

When Something Seems Off

"I may be missing something, but I'm noticing [specific observation]. Can the team take another look?"

"I may be missing something" is the magic phrase. It opens the door without coming in swinging.

When You Need a Different Plan

"I hear that, but [specific concern]. Is there another option we can consider?"

When You're Being Brushed Off

"I'd like to be sure this is documented. Can you note in the chart that I asked about [specific concern]?"

This usually gets immediate attention. Things in the chart matter.

When You Want to Slow Things Down

"Before we make this decision, I'd like a few minutes to talk it through with my family. Can we have 15 minutes?"

You are allowed to do this. You are allowed to ask for time. Especially for non-emergent decisions, this is a reasonable request.

The "Kind But Not Kidding" Posture

Here's the demeanor that works, in any setting:

- Eye contact, calm voice, even pace.

- Acknowledge them as humans: "I know you're slammed today. I just need a minute on this."
- State the concern clearly. One thing at a time.
- Ask a specific question.
- Wait for the answer. Don't fill the silence.
- If the answer doesn't satisfy you, say: "I hear that. I'm still concerned about [X]. Who else should I be talking to?"

I want to share something from the other side of this, because I think it matters.

As a nurse, manager, and administrator, I took a lot of calls from upset patients and family members. And most of the time? The concern was completely valid. The problem was the approach.

Some people came in swinging. Threats of violence. Promises to blast the facility on social media. Mentions of lawsuits in the first thirty seconds. Then there were the people who called and said something like: "Mom's medication was supposed to be called in yesterday but the pharmacy doesn't have it. Can you help us?"

Both calls got the same honest review of the concern and the fastest possible resolution. The outcome wasn't different based on how upset someone was — it was based on what the actual problem was and what we could do to fix it.

But the people who threatened violence? They often also received a discharge letter. Because healthcare workers are employees, not punching bags. They don't have to absorb threats, especially ones they didn't earn. Losing your care team in the middle of a medical crisis is the last thing you want.

Kindness is not weakness. The kindest people in the room are often the ones the staff respects most. They're also the ones who get their calls returned first.

When You Disagree With a Provider

It happens. Your gut says one thing, the doctor recommends another. Maybe the treatment plan feels too aggressive, or not aggressive enough. Maybe something about the discharge timeline doesn't sit right. Maybe you've done your research and you have real questions. Good. Ask them.

You are allowed to disagree. You are allowed to ask for a second opinion. You are allowed to slow down. Specifically:

- **Ask the question explicitly.** "I'd like to understand the reasoning here. Help me understand why this is the right choice."
- **Share your concern, not just your preference.** "I'm worried because last time she had this med, she had a bad reaction."
- **Ask for time.** "Is this something we have to decide today, or can we take 24 hours to think about it?"
- **Get a second opinion if it's a major decision.** Surgery, cancer treatment plans, end-of-life decisions — always reasonable to get another set of eyes. Most providers are not offended by this. The good ones welcome it.

If You're Being Treated Differently

Sometimes families experience providers who don't listen. And I want to be honest with you: this happens more to some people than others. Women get told their pain is anxiety. Older patients get told their symptoms are just aging. People of color are statistically less likely to have their pain taken seriously. Non-English-speaking patients get rushed through. If any of this is happening to your loved one — if real concerns are being dismissed or minimized — you are not imagining it. And you have options.

I'll never forget something I heard in a training years ago. A speaker shared that she had come across a term being used in some clinical settings to describe a middle-aged, pre- or menopausal woman who came in with concerns: "WWW." It stood for Whiny White Woman.

I want you to sit with that for a second. Because if that label exists for one group, you can bet variations of it exist for others.

If you feel like you're being ignored, looked over, or dismissed — get backup. Ask for another doctor. Ask for the patient advocate. You do not have to accept being minimized.

- **Document.** Specific words used, dates, names. Patterns matter.
- **Switch providers.** You are allowed. Find someone who listens.
- **Use a patient advocate.** Most hospitals and large practices have them.
- **File a complaint.** Especially if the dismissiveness leads to a missed diagnosis or harm.

When to Escalate

Most things get resolved at the first conversation. When they don't, here's the chain — in any setting:

In a Hospital

- Bedside nurse
- Charge nurse
- Nursing supervisor / nursing manager
- Hospitalist or attending physician
- Patient advocate / patient relations
- Administrator on Call
- Hospital ethics committee (for genuinely complex disagreements about care)

In a Clinic or Practice

- Medical assistant
- Triage nurse / nurse on duty
- Provider directly (often via patient portal)
- Office manager

- Department director or medical director (for larger systems)

With Insurance

- Member services rep
- Supervisor
- Case management
- Formal grievance / complaint
- State insurance commissioner (yes, you can complain there for genuinely wrong denials)

Don't skip steps unless you truly have to — going straight to the top before the lower levels have had a chance usually means coming back down anyway, with extra friction. But don't be afraid to climb either. These levels exist for a reason. Use them.

How to Frame a Complaint That Gets Action

If you ever need to escalate formally — to a patient advocate, an office manager, or in writing — structure it like this:

- The fact pattern (what happened, when, who was involved). Specific. Dated.
- The impact (what consequences this had, or could have).
- The request (what you want done).

Example:

"On April 14th, my mother was discharged from your facility with prescriptions for both Coumadin and Eliquis, two anticoagulants that should not be taken together. The discharging hospitalist was Dr. Smith. I caught the error at the pharmacy. I'd like a formal review of the discharge medication reconciliation process, and I'd like a written response to me about how this will be prevented."

That's a complaint a hospital takes seriously. It's specific, it cites the impact, and it asks for something tangible. Compare it to: "You guys are dangerous." Same anger, very different outcome.

Here's something worth saying out loud: by the time most people file a formal complaint, the damage is already done. You wouldn't be filing it otherwise. The point isn't to undo what happened — it's to make sure it doesn't happen again. To you, to your loved one, or to the next family who walks through those doors. That matters. Don't let anyone make you feel like complaining is petty. Done right, it's one of the most useful things you can do.

And let me tell you why filing that formal complaint is worth it, even when it feels exhausting.

When caring for Dave, we came across a provider who was arrogant, dismissive, and at times genuinely dangerous in his approach to patient care. I filed a formal complaint against him for something that happened during Dave's treatment. Everyone seemed to know about this provider — in passing conversations, people would shake their heads, say they didn't trust him, talk about things he had done. It was an open secret.

A year later I was with another loved one and we crossed paths with the same provider. Same attitude. Same demeaning arrogance. I filed another formal complaint on behalf of that family.

When the process was complete I found out something that stopped me cold: in all the time that provider had worked at that facility, only two formal complaints had ever been filed against him. Both of them were mine.

Everyone else had just talked about it. They complained to each other in hallways and waiting rooms and parking lots. But they never acted. And because they never acted, nothing changed.

If you encounter a provider who is unsafe, dismissive, or dangerous — please don't just talk about it. Act. File the complaint. Create the record. You may be the only one who does. And that record may be exactly what protects the next patient who doesn't have someone like you in their corner.

Do This Next

- **Memorize three scripts.** "I need clarification on..." "Can you explain why we're choosing this over..." "Can you note in the chart that I asked about..."
- **The next time something feels off, don't sit on it.** Speak up calmly, specifically, and to the right person. Use the chain.
- **Build a relationship with the bedside nurse or office MA** at your loved one's main practice. A name, a chat, a thank-you. These small things compound.
- **Practice the pause.** When the doctor says something that sounds like a decision, before you nod, take a breath and ask: "Can we slow down for a second — I want to make sure I understand?"
- **If you have a legitimate complaint, file it.** Don't just talk about it in the parking lot. Create the record. It may be the only one that exists.

In the next chapter, we get into the trickier territory: when something feels off, how do you know whether you're seeing what you think you're seeing? And what do you do about it?

Chapter Ten

When Something Feels Off (And What to Do About It)

Trust the Pit in Your Stomach

There is a particular feeling caregivers know. It's not panic. It's not anger. It's the quiet wrongness in your chest when you're standing next to your loved one's bed, or sitting in a clinic, or hanging up the phone after a call with a nurse, and something just isn't right.

Maybe Mom's medication was changed and you weren't told why. Maybe the doctor seemed dismissive when you mentioned the new symptom. Maybe Dad seems different today, and nobody's noticing. Maybe the discharge plan sounds great but the timing is wrong.

Whatever the specific shape of it, that feeling is data. Don't ignore it.

This chapter is about how to take that feeling seriously, sort it out, and act on it without spiraling — and without being dismissed.

Trusting Your Gut

Caregivers are usually the first to know when something is wrong. Not because they're medical experts, but because they're the people who actually know the patient. You know what your loved one looks like on a normal Tuesday. You know what their voice sounds like before a UTI starts. You know how they move, how they sleep, how they eat.

Healthcare workers don't have that baseline. They're working off a 12-hour shift's worth of observation. You have years.

This is why "she's just not herself" is a real clinical observation, even though it sounds vague. When a family says that to me as a nurse, I take it seriously. The good providers do. The thing is — you have to **say it.** Out loud. To the right person.

The wrongness in your chest doesn't make it into the chart unless you put it there.

What Actually Goes Wrong: The Real List

Most of the time, healthcare works. But when it doesn't, the failures tend to cluster in the same places. Knowing the patterns means you can watch for them.

Missed or Delayed Diagnoses

- **Symptoms attributed to the wrong cause.** "It's just anxiety." "It's just aging." Sometimes that's true. Sometimes it's a missed cardiac issue, thyroid problem, or cancer.
- **A test result that wasn't followed up on.** Labs come back abnormal. The provider was supposed to call. The call never came.
- **Multiple specialists, no quarterback.** Each one focused on their lane, nobody putting the whole picture together.

Medication Errors

- **Wrong dose.** Got a pill at the wrong strength. Especially common after hospital discharges.
- **Drug interactions.** New med added without checking what they were already on.
- **Duplicate prescriptions.** Both the old and new versions on the list. Patient takes both.
- **Wrong patient.** Rare in clinics, more common in hospitals. Always check the wristband and confirm the name.

Communication Breakdowns

- **Specialist didn't get the message** from the PCP, and vice versa.
- **Discharge instructions don't match what was said in the room.**
- **Different providers giving different answers** without anyone reconciling them.
- **Family member not informed** of important decisions or changes.

Bedside Care Issues

- **Pain not managed.** Patient says they're a 9, gets a 4-strength response.
- **Falls not prevented** when the patient is at obvious risk.
- **Pressure injuries** developing because someone wasn't being turned.
- **Infections.** Especially urinary or wound infections that weren't caught early.
- **Delirium not recognized.** Hospital-acquired delirium is extremely common in older patients and frequently gets dismissed as baseline behavior or "just confusion" — when it's actually a medical event that needs attention.

If any of these patterns sound familiar, you're not paranoid. They are common enough that any nurse with a few years of experience has seen them all.

What to Do in the Moment

When the gut feeling shows up — when you spot something that seems wrong — don't freeze and don't spiral. Here's the move.

- **Pause.** Don't react in your head. Look at the actual situation.
- **Get specific.** Translate the feeling into a fact. "She's confused" → "She doesn't know what year it is, and yesterday she did." "This seems wrong" → "This is the third med dose she's missed today."
- **Find the closest person who can act.** Bedside nurse, MA, on-call provider. Tell them the specific thing you noticed.
- **Ask one direct question.** "Can we get this checked? What's the next step?"
- **Document.** Note the time, the person you spoke with, what they said.
- **If it doesn't get addressed in a reasonable time, escalate.** Up the chain.

How to Document Concerns

Documentation is your friend. Three reasons: it forces clarity, it creates a record if things go wrong, and it gives you something to bring back to the conversation if you have to escalate.

A simple template:

Date / Time: 4/14/26, 2:15 p.m.

Who: Bedside nurse Sarah, charge nurse Mike

What I observed: Mom said her chest hurts — "a pressure feeling." Started about 30 minutes ago.

What I asked: Can we have this checked / can we get a doctor in to see her.

Response: Mike said the hospitalist was paged.

Follow-up: 2:45 p.m. — hospitalist Dr. Lee in room, ordered EKG and troponin.

Boring. Vital. If anything later goes wrong, this is what protects everyone — including the staff. They know it. They will respect families who keep good notes.

You don't need a special app or a fancy system. A spiral notebook and a pen work perfectly. The point is to write it down. And when you do — keep feelings out of it. You want facts only. Not "the nurse was dismissive and didn't seem to care." Instead: "I spoke with nurse Sarah at 2:15 p.m. and reported chest pain. She left the room without a response time or next step." One of those is a feeling. The other is a record. Only one of them helps you when it matters.

The Chain of Command

You saw the chain of command in the last chapter. The same logic applies here — start with the closest person who can act, work your way up, and don't skip steps unless the situation is urgent. If your loved one is in a skilled nursing facility, there's one addition worth knowing: every state has a Long-Term Care Ombudsman. This is a government-appointed advocate whose entire job is to investigate complaints about skilled nursing facilities and assisted living facilities. They are free, they are independent, and they have real authority. Find your state's Long-Term Care Ombudsman and bookmark the number before you need it.

When to Push Harder

Most of the time, calm and persistent gets the job done. But there are moments when calm isn't enough and waiting is dangerous. Here's when to stop being patient and start being loud.

- **A clinical change that's not being acted on.** New chest pain, sudden confusion, breathing changes, severe pain that's not being managed. If the bedside nurse hasn't moved in 15–30 minutes for an obvious clinical concern, ask for the charge nurse. If still nothing, ask for the hospitalist. For acute deterioration, ask if your hospital has a rapid response team you can request directly.

- **A pattern of being ignored.** You've raised the same concern three times to three different people. Time to go up: nursing supervisor, patient advocate.
- **A safety issue.** Falls, medication errors, neglect, suspected abuse. These are not "someday" concerns. Escalate today, in writing if needed.
- **A discharge that doesn't feel safe.** Use your appeal rights. If your loved one is on Medicare, the hospital is required by law to give you a document called the "Important Message from Medicare." It explains your right to appeal a discharge decision you disagree with. If you believe your loved one is being sent home too soon — medically unstable, no safe plan in place, equipment not ready — you can use this notice to formally appeal. The appeal review typically happens within 24 to 72 hours, and discharge is delayed while it's being reviewed. You do not have to accept a discharge you believe is unsafe. Read that notice the moment it's handed to you. If nobody has given it to you, ask for it by name. *(A current copy of the Important Message from Medicare is included in the Bonus Section at the back of this book.)*

When the Feeling Was Right

I want to tell you about a moment when trusting that feeling was the difference between catching something and missing it entirely.

You may remember from an earlier chapter that Dave ended up in the emergency department after his gamma knife procedure, when his brain began to swell. What I didn't tell you is what happened before the transfer.

The physician on duty — the same one I mentioned in the last chapter — tried to write off Dave's symptoms as a normal response to having a brain procedure the day before. He was calm about it.

Confident. He told me this was expected.

I knew better. I had spoken with Dave's radiation oncologist. According to him, Dave should have been able to return to work the next day. If he couldn't, something was wrong. I told the provider that directly. He shrugged it off.

When I pressed again, he told me that the MRI Dave had earlier that morning was fine — so his brain was fine.

We had been in that emergency room for hours. There had been no MRI that morning.

What he had pulled up was an MRI from a year earlier — one that happened to fall on the same date of the month. He had the wrong record. He was looking at old imaging and using it to dismiss a current emergency.

I pushed for a CT scan. We got it. We know how that turned out — the swelling was real, the transfer was necessary, and the intervention that followed mattered.

Before I left that facility, I filed a formal complaint.

Here is what I want you to take from this: I am a nurse and a healthcare administrator. I knew what questions to ask and what the answers should sound like. I had insider knowledge that most families don't have. And even with all of that, I was still dismissed — twice — before I got the right answer.

You may not have my background. But you have something just as important: you know your person. You know their baseline. You know what normal looks like for them. When something feels wrong, that knowledge is worth fighting for. Don't let anyone — no matter how confident they sound — talk you out of what you know.

When to Get a Second Opinion

If something major is being decided and something feels off — the diagnosis doesn't sit right, the treatment plan feels rushed, your gut is telling you to slow down — a second opinion is absolutely reasonable. This isn't about distrust or being difficult. It's about making sure you have the full picture before a major, potentially irreversible decision gets made.

You don't need a second opinion when you understand the plan, you trust the team, and the reasoning makes sense to you. But when any of these are true, ask:

- The diagnosis is unclear or surprising.
- The recommended treatment is invasive, irreversible, or has serious side effects and something feels off.
- You feel pressured to decide quickly.
- Multiple options exist and the trade-offs haven't been clearly explained.
- Your gut is telling you something isn't right.

Most insurance plans cover second opinions — but call and confirm before you go, so there are no surprises on the bill. Most providers are not offended by the request. If the first provider acts annoyed about it, that's data too — it's a sign their ego is at the wheel, and you may want that second opinion specifically because of how they reacted.

After the Fact: Reporting and Reviewing

Sometimes you don't catch something in the moment. You catch it later — in the car on the way home, or at 2 a.m., or when the bill arrives and something doesn't add up. A medication that shouldn't have been given. A fall that wasn't reported. A delay that mattered. It's not too late to act.

- **Request the medical records.** You have a right to them. Read what was documented.
- **File a formal complaint with the facility.** Patient relations or the hospital ombudsman.

- **File with the state.** Department of Health for hospital and SNF complaints. State licensing boards for individual provider complaints.
- **File with the hospital's accreditation organization.** Hospitals are accredited by outside organizations that take complaints seriously. The three most common are The Joint Commission (TJC), DNV GL (Det Norske Veritas), and OHFLAC — the Office of Healthcare Facility Licensure and Certification. There should be signage posted somewhere in the facility listing which accrediting body oversees them and how to contact them. You may also find this information in your admission packet. If you can't find it, ask the patient advocate.
- **Talk to a healthcare attorney** if there's a real injury. Not for revenge — for accountability and to make sure the same thing doesn't happen to someone else's mom.

Most caregivers don't pursue any of this, because they're exhausted. That's understandable. But if a real harm occurred and you can muster the energy, the system only changes when families speak up afterward.

A Note on Self-Doubt

After something goes wrong, caregivers often spiral into "I should have caught it sooner." Let me be plain: you are not the trained professional. You are not paid to know. You are doing this on top of jobs and kids and grief and exhaustion. The fact that you noticed at all is the win.

Catch what you can. Push when you can. Forgive yourself when you can't. The system has cracks. You are not the cause of them.

Do This Next

- **Print the documentation template** above and keep it in your notebook. Use it any time something feels off.
- **Save the patient advocate's number** for whatever facility

your loved one is most often in. You'd rather have it and not need it.

- **Practice the phrase: "She's just not herself, and I'm worried."** Say it out loud once. The next time you feel it, it'll come out easier.
- **Find out which accreditation organization oversees your loved one's facility and save the contact information.** Check the signage or the admission packet.
- **If you're ever handed the Important Message from Medicare, read it immediately.** Don't set it aside. Your window to act is short.

Next chapter — medications. The single biggest source of problems in caregiving, and the easiest to fix once you know how. Don't skip it.

Chapter Eleven

Medications, Lists, and Avoiding Mistakes

The Single Biggest Risk — and the Easiest to Manage

If you remember nothing else from this entire book, remember this: medications are where most of the preventable harm happens in healthcare. Not bad surgeons. Not missed diagnoses. Pills.

Wrong dose. Drug interactions. Duplicates. Stopped meds that should have been continued. Continued meds that should have been stopped. Medications that interact with new ones. Pills your loved one used to take but you forgot to mention. Vitamins that are actually messing with the blood thinner.

The good news is that medication problems are also the easiest thing to prevent. A simple list, kept current, in your hand at every appointment, will save your loved one's life or quality of life more than any other single thing you do in this entire book. So let's build it.

Why Medication Errors Happen

Knowing why this goes wrong helps you spot the moments when it's about to.

- **Multiple prescribers, no one in charge.** PCP adds something. Cardiologist adds something. ER adds something. Nobody talks. Mom is now on three medications that don't play well together.
- **Hospital discharges.** This is the highest-risk moment. New meds get added, old ones get stopped, doses change — and the discharge med list often doesn't match what was at home.
- **Look-alike, sound-alike drugs.** Hydroxyzine vs hydralazine. Metformin vs metronidazole. One letter, completely different drugs.
- **Confusing dose schedules.** "Take one tablet twice daily, except on Tuesdays" — nobody remembers.
- **Stopped taking it without telling anyone.** Usually because of side effects, cost, or because they felt better and figured they didn't need it anymore. Always call the prescriber before stopping anything.
- **OTCs and supplements.** Vitamins and herbal supplements are real drugs. They interact with prescriptions. People forget to mention them because they don't think of them as "meds."
- **Pharmacy mistakes.** Rare but real. Wrong pill in the bottle, wrong dose printed on the label.

There's also a clinical term worth knowing: **polypharmacy.** It refers to the use of multiple medications simultaneously — typically five or more — and it's one of the leading causes of medication errors, falls, confusion, and hospitalizations in older adults. If your loved one is seeing multiple specialists and the medication list keeps growing, it's worth asking the PCP directly: "Can we do a full medication review? I want to make sure everything on this list still needs to be here."

Every one of these is preventable, and the prevention is mostly the same: a clear, current list, and a habit of asking the right questions when anything changes.

The Master Medication List

This is the most important document in your binder. Make it. Keep it updated. Carry it everywhere.

What Goes On It

- **Drug name** — brand and generic if you know both (e.g., Eliquis / apixaban).
- **Dose** — the strength of each pill (e.g., 5 mg).
- **Frequency** — how often (twice daily, every morning, every 8 hours, etc.).
- **Route** — mouth, injection, inhaler, patch, etc.
- **What it's for** — in plain language. "Blood thinner" not "anticoagulant."
- **Who prescribed it** — PCP? Cardiologist?
- **Start date** — when they began taking it (if known).
- **Allergies and reactions** — a separate section. "Penicillin — hives in 1998."
- **Over-the-counter medications and supplements** — vitamins, herbals, antacids, fish oil, melatonin, anything they take regularly.

Print at least two copies. Keep one in the binder. Keep one in your bag. And take a photo of it with your phone. The paper might not be with you — your phone almost certainly will be. Update **every time something changes**, not someday when you have time.

Sample Format

Eliquis (apixaban) — 5 mg — twice daily — mouth — blood thinner for atrial fibrillation — Dr. Chen (Cardiology) — started 11/2024

That's it. One line per drug. Easy to scan. Easy to hand to a clinician.

Why This Matters: A Story From My Own Family

Let me tell you something that happened within a month of me writing this very section.

My mother called me — she's in her sixties, takes care of herself, pretty sharp — complaining that her doctor had changed her prescription for her "potassium" without telling her. They had apparently increased it from 50 to 100, and she wanted my help figuring out how to get her levels checked to see if she even needed the increase.

Something wasn't adding up. That didn't sound like a potassium dose. I couldn't even think of a clinical reason she'd be on straight potassium supplementation. So I told her what I'd tell anyone: call your provider. This doesn't make sense. Push back.

She argued with me for a beat — because that's just how we roll — but she called.

It turned out her "potassium" wasn't potassium at all. It was Losartan Potassium — the generic name for a blood pressure medication. She had her medications confused, didn't have a clear list, and had no idea what she was actually taking or why.

Her PCP did the right thing. They made her an appointment for the next day and required her to bring every single medication she had in the house. All of it. And they sorted her out. Or at least attempted to — but she's my mother, so I know exactly what that job is like.

This is why we make the list. Not just for the people we're caring for. For everyone. Including the people who insist they've got it handled.

The "Before Anything New" Questions

Any time a new medication is being prescribed — in a clinic, ER, or hospital — ask these questions before you walk out:

- **"What is this medication for?"** Plain English.
- **"How do we take it — how much, when, with food or**

without, and for how long?"

- **"Are there side effects we should watch for?"** Especially the ones that should make you call back.
- **"Are there any interactions with what they're already on?"** Hand them the list. Let them check.
- **"Is there a generic, and is it covered by insurance?"** Cost matters. Some brand names cost 20x the generic.
- **"Are we starting this in addition to anything, or replacing something?"** This is the question that catches duplicate prescriptions.
- **"If this isn't working, when do we follow up?"**

These seven questions take about 90 seconds. They prevent enormous problems.

A Note on Side Effects and Dr. Google

Every medication has a listed side effect profile, and most of them include the same usual suspects — nausea, vomiting, diarrhea, constipation. Before you spiral down a rabbit hole, ask yourself the most important question: is the side effect, if it even occurs, worse than what we're treating? If your loved one has been prescribed an inhaler to help them breathe and you read that it can cause nausea — which is the worse symptom? Most people would choose a little nausea over struggling to breathe. That is a decision you and your loved one have to make together.

And when you use Dr. Google, ChatGPT, or any other tool to research medications — and you will, and that's fine — remember that you get a response appropriate to the question you asked. If you're not asking the right question, you may not get the right answer. Use those tools to get informed, not to get scared. Then bring your real questions to the pharmacist or the provider.

Pharmacy vs Provider — Use Both

Pharmacists are wildly underused. They are drug experts. They have computer systems that flag interactions across all of your loved one's prescriptions — if (and this is important) **all the prescriptions are at the same pharmacy.**

One pharmacy. Always. Use one pharmacy for everything. Mail-order? Pick a brand and stick with it. CVS? All meds at CVS. The moment you split between pharmacies, you lose the safety net of someone seeing the whole picture.

If you use a mail-order pharmacy for maintenance medications, make sure your local pharmacy has a complete list of everything being filled by mail. The safety net only works if someone can see the whole picture.

If you have a med question and the doctor's office is closed or slow, call the pharmacy first. They can answer dose questions, side effect questions, interaction questions, whether it's safe to take with food or alcohol or another OTC, and what to do if a dose was missed. And they don't charge for the call. Use them.

Reconciliation During Transitions

Every time your loved one moves between settings — hospital to home, hospital to rehab, rehab to home, home to ER and back — the medication list needs to be reconciled. "Reconciled" means someone sits down with both lists — what they were taking before, and what's prescribed now — compares them line by line, and explains every single difference. Added, stopped, changed, and why.

This is the moment things go wrong most often. The hospital adds three new meds. They miss that one of them is a duplicate of a med Mom was already on. They send her home with both. She takes both. Now she's bleeding from the GI tract.

Your job at every transition: get the discharge medication list in writing. Compare it line by line to the home medication list. Anything different, ask: "Why is this changed?"

The Transition Med Reconciliation Routine

- **Get the home list out** before discharge.
- **Get the discharge list** before they hand you papers.
- **Compare them.** Three columns: home / new / explanation.
- **For each change, ask:** "Is this stopped, started, or changed? Why?"
- **Confirm out loud:** "So at home today she'll take A, B, C, and the new D. She is no longer taking E and F. Is that right?"
- **Get the new prescriptions filled.** Check the pharmacy label against the discharge list when you pick up. Same drug, same dose, same frequency? If not, call back.

Common Caregiver Med Mistakes

Things I see all the time, in case any of these are happening at your house:

- **Mixing up morning and evening meds** because they look similar. → Use a pill organizer with morning/evening compartments.
- **Forgetting whether a dose was given today.** → Use a checkbox sheet or an organizer that shows the current day.
- **Stopping a medication because of a side effect, without telling anyone.** → Always call the prescriber. Some side effects fade. Some medications can't be stopped abruptly without harm.
- **Splitting pills that aren't supposed to be split.** → Some are scored and split fine. Some are extended-release and splitting destroys the dosing. Ask the pharmacist.
- **Storing meds in the bathroom.** Heat and humidity degrade medications faster than most people realize — and bathrooms are the worst possible place for them despite what everyone does. Store in a cool, dry place like a bedroom dresser or kitchen cabinet away from the stove.

- **Giving the wrong person's medication by accident.** When multiple people in a household are on medications, especially if pill organizers are being used, it's easier than you'd think to grab the wrong one. Label everything clearly. Keep different people's medications in completely separate locations.
- **Skipping doses to save money — or convenience.** Talk to the pharmacist about cost — there are often patient assistance programs, manufacturer coupons, or generic alternatives. But skipping doses for convenience is just as common and just as dangerous.

Here's a real example of why convenience skipping backfires:

Lasix — also called furosemide — is a diuretic, commonly known as a "fluid pill." It helps the body remove excess fluid, and it's prescribed daily for a reason. People skip it all the time because they don't want to be running to the bathroom when they have somewhere to go. Here's the problem: skipping a dose doesn't make the fluid go away. It just lets it build up. Then when you take it the next day, your body is now clearing two days' worth of retained fluid — so you end up going to the bathroom more than you would have if you'd just taken it consistently. You created the exact problem you were trying to avoid.

The fix is simple: take it first thing in the morning. It does its job while you're home, and by the time you need to go anywhere, you're fine. Ask your provider or pharmacist about timing — for many medications, when you take it matters just as much as whether you take it.

Tools That Actually Help

- **Weekly pill organizer** with morning/noon/evening/bedtime compartments. The single best $10 you'll spend.
- **A second pill organizer** for two-week travel or hospital stays.
- **A med list app** like Medisafe or your pharmacy's app, if you'll actually use one. Reminders matter.
- **Phone alarms** with the name of the med in the alarm label.

Beats relying on memory.

- **A fridge note** with the current med list and any "as needed" guidance. This one is more important than it sounds — first responders and emergency medical technicians are trained to check the refrigerator door for medication lists when they respond to a call. If your loved one ever needs emergency help and can't speak for themselves, that list on the fridge could be the first thing the paramedics see.

"As Needed" (PRN) Medications — Use With Care

PRN is a Latin abbreviation — pro re nata — that means "as needed." You'll see it on labels for pain meds, anti-anxiety medications, sleep aids, and nausea medications. "As needed" sounds simple. It isn't always.

- **Know the maximum dose per day.** "Take 1 every 4 hours as needed for pain, not to exceed 4 per day." Write it on the label if you have to.
- **Know what counts as "as needed."** Some people start using PRN meds daily. That's not what "as needed" means. If your loved one is taking it daily, the prescription should be revisited.
- **Watch for acetaminophen.** Acetaminophen — sold as Tylenol — is hiding in more medications than most people realize. Cold medicines, sleep aids, combination pain relievers like oxycodone/acetaminophen and hydrocodone/acetaminophen. It is very easy to accidentally take too much without knowing it. Always check the label of every OTC medication for acetaminophen before giving it to someone already taking Tylenol or a combination prescription.

For a healthy adult, the maximum recommended dose of acetaminophen is 4,000 mg per day — though many providers recommend staying under 3,000 mg to be safe. For someone with liver disease, chronic alcohol use, or other liver concerns, that limit drops significantly — often to 2,000 mg per day or less. When in doubt, ask the pharmacist. This is exactly the kind of question they are there for.

- **Watch for ibuprofen interactions.** Ibuprofen interacts with blood thinners and can be hard on the kidneys. Always check before giving it alongside other medications.

Reading the Pharmacy Label

Every prescription label has the same parts. Knowing them helps catch errors when you pick up.

- **Patient name** — confirm it's correct.
- **Drug name and strength** — e.g., Lisinopril 10 mg.
- **Quantity** — how many pills in the bottle.
- **Sig** — short for the Latin "signa," meaning instructions. This is the directions: "take 1 tablet by mouth daily." If anything here doesn't match what the provider told you in the office, ask before you leave the counter.
- **Refills** — how many remain.
- **Prescriber** — who ordered it.
- **Pharmacy phone** — in case there's a problem.

The first three minutes after you pick up a prescription is when you should compare the label to the discharge list. Mistakes are easier to fix at the counter than from your kitchen at 8 p.m.

Cost: When Meds Are Too Expensive

Plenty of caregivers face a moment when a prescription comes back at $400 a month and they stand at the pharmacy counter not knowing what to say. Don't walk out. Don't skip it and figure it out later. Say something right there. Here's what you can do:

- Ask the pharmacist for a generic.
- Ask the pharmacist about discount programs — GoodRx, manufacturer coupons, the pharmacy's own discount program.
- Call the prescriber to ask if there's a covered alternative.
- Ask about patient assistance programs — most expensive

drugs have manufacturer programs that can dramatically reduce cost for people who qualify.

- For Medicare patients, look at "Extra Help" — the federal program that helps with Part D costs.

Do This Next

- **Build the master medication list this week.** Print two copies. One in the bag, one on the fridge. Take a photo for your phone.
- **Pick one pharmacy** and consolidate everything there.
- **Buy a weekly pill organizer.** Use it. Refill it Sundays.
- **Save the seven "before anything new" questions** in your phone.
- **At the next transition** (hospital, ER, rehab, anywhere), do the reconciliation routine: home list, new list, line by line.

That's Part 3. You now know how to advocate, when something feels off, and how to manage the single biggest risk in healthcare. Up next: money. Bills, EOBs, and the charges nobody can explain. Bring coffee.

Chapter Twelve

Bills, Statements, and "What the Hell Is This Charge?"

How to Read a Medical Bill Without Throwing Up

You open the mail. There's an envelope from a hospital. You weren't expecting one. You open it. There's a number on it that ends in three zeros. Your hand starts to shake.

Take a breath. I am going to tell you something that has saved me, my family, and more people than I can count a lot of money: **do not pay the first thing that arrives in the mail.** Half of those documents aren't bills. The other half are wrong about a third of the time.

This chapter is about the paperwork side of healthcare — what each piece is, what to actually look at, and when not to pay yet.

Bill vs EOB — Know the Difference

There are two pieces of paper that look almost identical and mean completely different things. People mix them up constantly. Once you can tell them apart, half your stress goes away.

EOB — Explanation of Benefits

An EOB comes from **insurance.** It is **not a bill.** Right at the top, in big letters, it usually says: **THIS IS NOT A BILL.**

An EOB explains: this is what the provider charged, this is what insurance allowed, this is what insurance paid, this is what you may owe. It's a summary. It's information. It's not asking for money.

If you've signed up for paperless billing through your insurance company, your EOBs may arrive by email or be posted to your online account instead of showing up in the mail. Either way, the same rules apply — it is not a bill, and you should review it before any actual bill arrives.

Bill

A bill comes from the **provider** (the doctor's office, hospital, lab, imaging center). It says: this is what you owe, please pay by this date, here's how.

Critical: the EOB usually comes first. The actual bill follows, days or weeks later. So when an EOB shows up, your job is to understand it. Not to pay it. The bill comes next, and that is the document you actually compare and act on.

Charged vs Allowed vs Paid — The Three Numbers That Confuse Everyone

Every medical service has three numbers attached to it. Once you understand them, the EOB stops being terrifying.

- **Charged amount.** The provider's sticker price — and largely a fictional number. Hospitals set these rates high because insurance companies negotiate them down. Nobody with insurance actually pays the charged amount. It's the starting point for a negotiation that already happened before you walked in the door. And even if you're self-pay — meaning you have no insurance — you don't pay this number either. Self-pay patients are typically offered a discount automatically, and if you can pay in full, you can often negotiate an even bigger reduction. Never assume the charged amount is what you actually owe. It almost never is.

- **Allowed amount.** The negotiated rate between insurance and the provider. This is the real price. If insurance allows $1,200, that's what the procedure actually costs under your plan.
- **Paid amount + patient responsibility.** Of the allowed amount, insurance pays a portion, and you pay the rest (deductible, coinsurance, copay). The total of those two should equal the allowed amount.

Plain example, on an EOB:

Charged: $5,000 Allowed: $1,200 Insurance paid: $960 You owe: $240

That "you owe $240" is what should match the bill. If the bill says you owe more than the EOB says, that's a red flag and you need to call billing.

Why Bills Don't Match Expectations

There are a few common reasons bills come in surprising:

- **The deductible wasn't met yet.** Insurance "paid" $0 because nothing was covered until you hit the deductible. You owe the full allowed amount — not the charged amount, but the allowed amount. This is not a mistake. It's how insurance math works. Check where you are in your deductible year before you call billing confused.
- **Out-of-network provider.** Even at an in-network hospital, individual providers — anesthesiologists, radiologists, pathologists — bill separately from the facility. You can receive a bill from these

providers even when everything else was in-network. If those providers happen to be out-of-network, you'll be responsible for the out-of-network rate, which is typically significantly higher. Always check who was involved in your loved one's care and whether each provider is in-network — not just the hospital itself.

- **Surprise bill / balance bill.** When an out-of-network provider charges you the difference between what they billed and what insurance paid. Federal law (the No Surprises Act) limits this in many situations — see below.
- **Service wasn't covered.** Insurance denied something. Now you owe the full allowed (or charged) amount.
- **Coding error.** The wrong procedure code was used, or a diagnosis code was missing. Insurance denied. The bill came to you. This is fixable — the provider can correct and resubmit.
- **Bundled vs unbundled charges.** Sometimes services that should be billed as a bundle get billed individually, inflating the total.

How to Read a Medical Bill

Pull out the next bill that arrives. We're going to walk through it together.

- **Top-line info.** Patient name. Account number. Service date. Provider/facility name.
- **Date(s) of service.** When the care happened.
- **Description of services.** This is where the line items live. Each one has a CPT code — a five-digit number that represents a specific medical service or procedure — and a brief description. If a charge looks unfamiliar, the CPT code is what you use to look it up or ask about it. "Can you tell me what CPT code 99213 represents?" is a completely reasonable question to ask billing. If your bill doesn't list CPT codes or you can't make sense of the line items, call the facility and ask for an itemized bill. You have a right to one. The itemized

version breaks down every single charge individually — and that's often where errors show up that the summary bill hides.

- **Charges.** The fictional sticker price.
- **Adjustments / contractual adjustments.** What got knocked off because of the contract with insurance.
- **Insurance payments.** What insurance paid.
- **Patient responsibility / amount due.** What you owe.
- **Due date.** When they want it paid.
- **Payment options.** How to pay (online, mail, phone).

What to Question

Before you pay a single dollar, run the bill through these questions. This is not being difficult. This is being a smart consumer. The billing department expects these calls. They get them every day.

- **Did this service actually happen?** It sounds silly, but bills sometimes include things that didn't occur, especially during long hospital stays. Check your notes.
- **Is the date right?** Wrong date can mean wrong patient or duplicate billing.
- **Does the bill match the EOB?** Pull up the EOB for the same date of service. The patient responsibility on the bill should match the patient responsibility on the EOB.
- **Are there duplicate charges?** Same line item, same date, billed twice.
- **Was insurance billed?** If "insurance pending" or "self-pay" shows up on a bill for someone with insurance, something went wrong. Call before paying.
- **Were any services unexpectedly out-of-network?** If so, you may have rights under the No Surprises Act.
- **Are the codes right?** Sometimes a wrong code on the provider side leads to a denial that wasn't actually warranted. The

provider can correct and resubmit.

When NOT to Pay Yet

Hold off on paying when:

- **The EOB hasn't shown up yet.** Wait for the EOB. Compare to the bill.
- **The bill is dated within 30 days of the service.** Insurance often hasn't finished processing yet. It's very common for a bill to arrive before insurance has paid their portion. Wait for the EOB. The balance often drops significantly — or disappears entirely — once insurance settles.
- **The bill says "insurance pending" or "self-pay" when you have insurance.** Call. Get it corrected.
- **You see something that looks wrong.** Charges you don't recognize, services that didn't happen, an amount that doesn't match the EOB. Call before paying.
- **You haven't received the itemized bill.** What you got might be a summary. You have a right to a full itemized statement — ask for it. The detailed version often reveals errors.

Important: not paying yet is different from ignoring it. Always call the billing department, document the call, and note what they tell you — the date, the time, the name of the person you spoke with, and what they said. The facility should be documenting these calls on their end as well, but don't rely on that alone. Your notes are your protection. Set a reminder to follow up. Bills that go ignored end up in collections.

The No Surprises Act (Know This One)

Here's a law that exists specifically to protect you, and most people have never heard of it. The No Surprises Act, passed in 2022, limits what providers can charge you for out-of-network care in several specific situations:

- **Emergency services from out-of-network providers** (you

can only be charged in-network rates).

- **Out-of-network providers at in-network facilities** (anesthesiologists, radiologists, etc.) without your written consent.
- **Air ambulance services.**

If you get a bill that looks like it might be a surprise out-of-network bill, push back. The law applies. You may not actually owe the higher amount.

There's also a "good-faith estimate" requirement for self-pay patients (uninsured or paying out of pocket). If your final bill is more than $400 above the estimate, you can dispute it.

Why Questioning Bills Matters: A Story From After Dave

I want to share a story that happened after Dave passed away, because it illustrates exactly why you question every bill — even when you're exhausted, even when the amount seems small, even when you're in the middle of grief.

When someone passes, the estate is required to publish a notice in the local paper so that anyone owed a debt can make a claim. I received several bills from the local hospital during that process. Most were small — $25, $50. But one was somewhere between $100 and $200, and something about it didn't sit right. It showed that insurance had paid nothing on it, and it was from later in the year.

Here's what I knew: with Dave's cancer treatments, PET scans, and everything else, we hit our out-of-pocket maximum almost every year by January. That meant for the rest of the year, covered services were paid at 100% by insurance. So why was insurance paying nothing on a bill from later in the year?

I called. I pushed. I asked questions.

What I found out was that the charge had been coded under something called provider-based billing — a method that separates the facility fee from the professional fee and bills them independently.

Our insurance didn't reimburse under provider-based billing. They required what's called global billing, where all charges are submitted together in a single bill. The coding was wrong. The claim had been processed incorrectly. And because of that error, insurance had paid nothing — and we were being asked to cover it.

We didn't owe that money. Not a dollar of it.

I only caught it because something felt off and I asked. A grieving widow, dealing with an estate, looking at a bill that most people would have just paid and moved on. Please don't be most people.

Negotiating Hospital Bills

If you genuinely owe a balance you can't pay in full — or even if you can but it's a hardship — know this: hospital bills are negotiable. Most hospitals will not advertise this. You have to ask. And asking works.

- **Ask for the financial assistance application.** Nonprofit hospitals (most of them) are required to have one. If you qualify by income, the bill can be reduced significantly — sometimes wiped out.
- **Ask for a self-pay discount.** Even without qualifying for financial assistance, hospitals will sometimes knock 20–40% off if you pay in a lump sum.
- **Ask for a payment plan.** Often interest-free. "I can pay $50 a month" is a real option.
- **Compare the bill to fair-market prices.** Under federal price transparency rules, hospitals are required to publish their prices in a way that is easy for consumers to find on their website. You can also use tools like Valenz Bluebook (formerly Healthcare Bluebook) or FAIR Health Consumer to see what a service typically costs in your area. Use that information as leverage when negotiating.

This works. Many people have walked into a hospital billing office expecting a fight and walked out with a 50% reduction or a long-term payment plan.

If a Bill Goes to Collections

Sometimes a bill ends up in collections by mistake — insurance was still processing, the bill went to the wrong address, or it got lost in the chaos of caregiving. It happens more than you'd think, and it doesn't mean you did something wrong. Take a breath. Medical debt has more protections than most other kinds of debt, and you have options.

- **Send a written request for verification of the debt.** They are legally required to provide it.
- **Check the dates.** If the bill is wrong, dispute it in writing.
- **Try to settle directly with the provider** if it's still possible — they often pull it back from collections.
- **For active dispute, you can ask for the debt to be removed pending resolution.** As of recent rule changes, paid medical collections under $500 are no longer reported to credit bureaus, and some others have longer reporting waits. Worth knowing.

Keeping the Paperwork Sane

A simple system that works for most caregivers:

- **One folder for EOBs,** sorted by date.
- **One folder for bills,** sorted by date.
- **One running spreadsheet or notebook page** with: date of service, provider, amount billed, amount paid, status.
- **One sticky note rule:** if it looks scary, don't pay until you've called once.

If you prefer to go digital, the same system works — one folder on your computer or cloud storage for EOB PDFs, one for bills, and a simple spreadsheet to track everything. Either way, the goal is the same: when a bill arrives, you should be able to find the matching EOB in under two minutes.

Scripts for Calling Billing

To Get Clarity on a Bill

"Hi, I'm calling about a bill for [Name], account number [#], date of service [date]. The amount is $X. I'm trying to understand the charges — can you walk me through them, and confirm whether insurance has finished processing?"

To Question a Specific Charge

"I'm looking at a charge for [item] on [date], for $X. I don't see this on the EOB — can you explain what this is and confirm it was billed to insurance?"

To Dispute a Charge

"I've reviewed this bill against my EOB and I believe there may be an error. The EOB shows my patient responsibility as $X, but this bill shows $Y. Before I make any payment, I'd like this reviewed and corrected if needed. Can you open a review and give me a reference number for this call?"

To Ask for Financial Assistance

"I received a bill for $X. I don't have the means to pay this in full. Do you have a financial assistance program, and can you send me the application? I'd also like to know my options for a payment plan in the meantime."

To Ask for a Self-Pay Discount

"If I were able to pay this in a lump sum, what discount could you offer?"

Do This Next

- **Set up two folders — EOBs and Bills** — and sort what you have.
- **Make a one-page spreadsheet** of services and charges to track what you've paid, what you owe, and what's still pending.
- **Adopt the rule:** EOB before bill, bill compared to EOB, call before paying anything that doesn't match.
- **Bookmark the No Surprises Act resources** at cms.gov/no

surprises so you have a reference if something looks fishy.

- **Save the financial assistance phone number** for any hospital your loved one uses regularly. You'd rather have it and not need it.

Up next: when insurance says no. Denials, appeals, and how to actually win.

Chapter Thirteen

Denials, Appeals, and Fighting Back

How to Read a Denial Letter Without Crying — and How to Win

If your loved one has spent any real time in the healthcare system, you've gotten a denial letter. Maybe a procedure denied as "not medically necessary." Maybe a medication denied because of "step therapy." Maybe a SNF stay denied after the first week. Maybe a flat-out "this service is not covered."

Here's what nobody tells you: **a large percentage of denials get reversed when families appeal.** Estimates vary, but for some categories of denials, more than half get overturned on appeal. The system is built on the assumption that most people will give up. The people who don't, win disproportionately often.

This chapter is going to teach you how to read a denial, how to appeal it, and how to actually win.

Why Insurance Denies Things

Before you can fight a denial, you need to know what kind of denial you're dealing with. Most fall into one of these buckets — and each one has a different fix.

- **Not medically necessary.** This is the most common denial reason. Insurance's medical reviewer looked at what was submitted and decided the documentation didn't meet their criteria to justify the service. It doesn't mean the service isn't needed — it means the paperwork didn't make the case strongly enough. This is very often fixable.
- **Lack of prior authorization.** A service that required advance approval from insurance was performed without it — or the authorization request was never submitted, or it expired before the service happened. Sometimes this is the provider's error, not yours.
- **Step therapy / formulary issues.** Insurance requires patients to try a cheaper medication first and have it fail before approving a more expensive one. This is called "fail first" or step therapy. Your doctor may know the cheaper option won't work — but insurance wants documented proof of that before they'll approve the alternative.
- **Out-of-network.** The provider or facility isn't in your plan's network, so insurance either won't cover it or covers it at a much lower rate. Sometimes this is a surprise — you went to an in-network hospital but one of the providers treating you wasn't in-network.
- **Service excluded under the plan.** Some services simply aren't covered — cosmetic procedures, certain experimental treatments, some forms of long-term care. If it's listed as an exclusion in your plan documents, this is the hardest denial to overturn.
- **Coding errors.** The wrong procedure code or diagnosis code was used, or two codes don't align the way insurance expects. This is a paper problem, not a clinical one, and it's usually fixable by having the provider's office correct and resubmit.
- **Eligibility issues.** Insurance lapsed, the wrong subscriber

information was submitted, or there's a plan year mismatch. Call insurance and the provider's billing office together to sort this out.

- **Coordination of benefits issues.** Your loved one has two insurance plans and they're disputing which one pays first. This is a bureaucratic tangle but it's solvable — both insurers need to talk to each other and establish who's primary.

How to Read a Denial Letter

Denial letters are intimidating. They're meant to be. Read them with this structure in mind.

- **Find the date of service.** What was being denied?
- **Find the reason for denial.** Usually one or two sentences, often with a code. "Reason: not medically necessary per InterQual criteria." Or "Reason: pre-authorization not on file."
- **Find the appeal rights section.** This is the most important part of the entire letter. It tells you the deadline — usually 60 to 180 days — where to send the appeal, and what kind of appeal it is. The moment you find this section, write the deadline on your calendar. Do it before you do anything else. A late appeal is an automatic loss regardless of how strong your case is.
- **Note the appeal type.** Is this a first-level appeal? An expedited appeal (faster, for urgent cases)? A standard appeal? Each has its own timeline.
- **Note any reference numbers** — case numbers, claim numbers. You'll need them on every call.

Read the letter twice. The first read for the gut punch. The second read for the actual information.

How to Appeal (Step by Step)

Step 1: Don't Wait

Appeals have deadlines. Often 60 days for commercial insurance. Sometimes longer for Medicare. Mark the deadline on the calendar the day the letter arrives. Do not procrastinate. The single biggest reason appeals fail is that they get filed late.

Step 2: Get the Records

You need to know what insurance saw when they denied. Two requests:

- **From the provider:** the office visit notes, lab results, imaging reports — anything that supports medical necessity.
- **From insurance:** the criteria they used to evaluate, the case notes, and the name and credentials of the reviewer who denied. Yes, you can request this — and you should. Knowing exactly what criteria they applied tells you precisely what your appeal needs to address.

Step 3: Loop In the Provider

This is the most important move and the one most people skip.

Call the provider's office and tell them about the denial. Ask: **"Can you do a peer-to-peer review with the insurance reviewer?"**

A peer-to-peer is a phone call between the doctor who ordered the service and the insurance company's medical director. It often resolves denials in a single 15-minute call. Insurance companies have to offer this. The provider has to be willing. Many denials get reversed at this step before a formal appeal is even necessary.

If the provider's office hesitates, push kindly but firmly: "I know it takes time. Can we please try? A 15-minute phone call could mean the difference between approval and a lengthy formal appeal process."

Step 4: Write the Appeal

If the peer-to-peer doesn't resolve it, or if the provider can't do one, file a formal written appeal. The structure that wins:

- **Patient identifier line at the top.** Name, DOB, member ID, claim number, denial date.
- **One-paragraph summary** of what was denied and why.
- **Why the denial is wrong** — specifically, addressing the rea-

son given. If they said "not medically necessary," this is where you cite the clinical reasoning.

- **Supporting documentation.** Provider letter, chart notes, lab results, relevant guidelines from professional societies (American Heart Association, American College of Physicians, etc., depending on the issue).
- **Specific request.** "We request that you reverse the denial and approve the [specific service]."
- **Contact info** for follow-up.

Keep it factual. Keep it specific. Avoid emotional language. The reviewer is not your enemy — they're a person reading 50 appeals a day. Make their job easy. Show them clearly why this case meets criteria.

Step 5: Submit and Track

- **Submit by the method the letter specifies** (often mail, fax, or online portal). If by mail, send certified with return receipt.
- Keep a copy of everything you send.
- **Note the date of submission** and the expected response timeline (usually 30 days standard, 72 hours expedited).
- **Follow up at the deadline.** If you haven't heard back, call. If they say they didn't receive it, you have proof.

Step 6: If the First Appeal Fails

Most plans have multiple levels of appeal:

- **First-level (internal) appeal** — reviewed by the insurance company.
- **Second-level (internal) appeal** — still inside the company, but typically reviewed by someone different.
- **External review** — an independent third party reviews the case. This is required by law for most denials. Many cases get overturned at external review.

Don't stop at the first no. The structure is built for multiple rounds. Going to external review is your right. Use it.

When One Phone Call Was All It Took

Let me give you an example of how simple this can sometimes be.

Years ago I had knee surgery. Not from an accident, not from an injury — just my body being my body. When the claim was processed, I received a denial. Insurance had determined the surgery was the result of an accident and denied it on that basis.

It wasn't an accident. There was no accident. I called insurance, explained that clearly, and they covered it.

That's it. One phone call. A denial reversed because the information they had was wrong and I took five minutes to correct it.

I share this because I want you to understand something: not every denial is a fight. Some are paperwork errors. Some are assumptions that were never verified. Some fall apart the moment someone calls and says "that's not right." The ones that do require a real fight — the formal appeals, the peer-to-peer reviews, the letter writing — those are worth fighting too. But start with the phone call. You might be surprised how often that's all it takes.

What Actually Increases Approval Chances

Not every appeal is created equal. The ones that win tend to share these features:

- **Filed on time.** Always. Late = automatic loss.
- **Includes a peer-to-peer attempt.** This step alone resolves many cases.
- **Includes a letter of medical necessity** from the ordering provider, addressed specifically to the denial reason.
- **Cites clinical guidelines.** From specialty societies, from the insurer's own published criteria, from FDA labels.
- **Documents prior conservative treatments tried.** If insur-

ance denied an MRI for back pain, evidence that physical therapy and medications were tried first is gold.

- **Includes patient and family statements.** Especially in functional terms — not "Mom is very sick" but "Mom can no longer walk to the bathroom without assistance and falls twice a week without the equipment being requested." The reviewers are humans. Specific, concrete, functional descriptions of impact carry real weight. One paragraph, in plain language, from someone who sees the patient every day.
- **Goes to external review when needed.** Many people stop at the second internal denial. The external reviewer is a different game.

When to Involve the Provider

Always. Truly. The provider's office can:

- Do the peer-to-peer review.
- Write a letter of medical necessity.
- Add additional clinical documentation.
- Resubmit with corrected codes if it was a coding error.
- Sometimes call insurance with you on a three-way line, which is occasionally what cracks the case.

The catch: provider offices are busy. Some have a dedicated appeals/PA team; some don't. Be polite, be patient, and be persistent. The squeaky (but kind) wheel gets the grease.

If the provider's office genuinely won't engage with the appeals process, that's important information. It may mean it's time to find a provider who will advocate for their patients. A doctor who isn't willing to spend 15 minutes on a peer-to-peer call for a service they ordered is worth noting.

Special Situations

Medicare Denials

Medicare has its own appeals process. Five levels, formally structured:

- Redetermination by the original Medicare contractor.
- Reconsideration by a Qualified Independent Contractor.
- Hearing before an Administrative Law Judge.
- Review by the Medicare Appeals Council.
- Federal court review.

Most cases don't go beyond level 2 or 3. The deadlines are tight (often 60 to 120 days at each level). The process is more formal but also more documented — every step has clear paperwork.

Hospital Discharge Denials

If Medicare denies coverage of additional hospital days because they think discharge is appropriate, you have the right to a fast appeal — within hours. The hospital must give you the "Important Message from Medicare" explaining how. Use it if you genuinely believe the discharge is unsafe.

SNF Denials

If a skilled nursing facility tells you Medicare won't cover any more days, you can appeal. The facility is required to give you a document called the Notice of Medicare Non-Coverage — sometimes called the NOMNC. This is your formal notification and your starting point for the appeal process. The first step is to contact the Quality Improvement Organization (QIO) for your state. Don't let the NOMNC sit. The window to act is short.

Medication / Formulary Denials

Often resolved by:

- **Step therapy override** — your doctor documents why the cheaper drug won't work.
- **Formulary exception request** — asking insurance to cover a drug not on their preferred list.
- **Tier exception** — asking for a drug to be covered at a lower

cost-sharing tier than its default tier.

Each has a specific form. Ask the pharmacy or insurance which applies.

If the formulary appeal doesn't go your way, don't give up on the medication entirely. Most expensive brand-name drugs have manufacturer patient assistance programs that can provide the medication at low or no cost for people who qualify. Ask the prescriber's office or go directly to the manufacturer's website.

If You're Stuck

Sometimes you do everything right and you still hit a wall. The appeal was filed on time. The provider wrote the letter. The peer-to-peer happened. And insurance still said no. That's not the end. Here are resources most families never know exist — and some of them are free, independent, and surprisingly powerful.

- **State insurance commissioner.** They take complaints. Sometimes a complaint here gets a denial reversed faster than another internal appeal.
- **State Health Insurance Assistance Program (SHIP).** Free Medicare counseling. Every state. They are a goldmine.
- **Patient advocacy nonprofits.** Many disease-specific organizations (cancer, kidney, etc.) have appeals support staff who do this for a living and will help free.
- **Healthcare attorneys** — typically last resort, but useful for high-stakes denials with significant cost.
- **Your employer's HR department.** If the insurance is through work, HR can sometimes apply pressure that an individual cannot.

Sample Appeal Letter Skeleton

Here is a starting point. Copy it, customize it, and make it specific to your situation. **A generic appeal loses. A specific one wins.**

Re: Appeal of Denial — [Patient Name], DOB [date], Member ID [#], Claim/Reference [#]

Date of Service: [date]

Denial Date: [date]

To Whom It May Concern,

I am writing to formally appeal the denial of [service or medication] for [patient name] dated [date]. The denial reason given was [exact wording from letter].

This denial is incorrect for the following reasons:

1. [Specific clinical reason. Reference the chart notes, lab results, prior treatments tried.]

2. [Citation to clinical guidelines or insurer's own criteria, if applicable.]

3. [Functional impact on the patient.]

Enclosed please find:

• Letter of medical necessity from [provider name]

• Office visit notes from [date]

• Lab/imaging results from [date]

• Prior treatment records

I request that the denial be reversed and [service] be approved.

Please contact me at [phone] or [email] with any questions.

Sincerely,

[Your name]

[Relationship to patient]

Do This Next

- **The next time you get a denial, write the appeal deadline on your calendar within 24 hours.** Don't wait. Don't rationalize. Mark it.
- **Save the appeal letter skeleton above.** Use it as a starting point. Customize for each case.

- **Call the provider before you write a single appeal letter.** Ask for a peer-to-peer. This single step solves a lot of denials.
- **Look up your state's insurance commissioner's website.** Bookmark the consumer complaint form.
- **Look up your state's SHIP program and save the number.** Free Medicare counseling, every state. Use it before you spend money on anything else.
- **For Medicare, bookmark Medicare.gov/claims-appeals.** It walks through every level.

That's Part 4. The boring, expensive part. You now have the tools to push back when you're told no. Up next: the part of caregiving nobody really prepares you for. The human side.

Chapter Fourteen

The Emotional Reality of Caregiving

The Emotional Reality of Caregiving

The Part Nobody Warns You About

If you've made it this far, you have learned a lot of practical things. How to organize information. How to advocate. How to read an EOB. How to appeal a denial. The mechanics.

This chapter is about something else. The part nobody warns you about. The part that hits you at 2 a.m. when the pump finally stops beeping and you can't sleep. The part that makes you cry in a Walmart parking lot over something small. The part that makes you snap at the people who love you, then feel guilty about it for three days.

This chapter is about the emotional reality of caregiving — told without bullshit, without inspirational quotes, and without the tidy resolution Hollywood likes.

Buckle up. We're going in.

The Exhaustion Nobody Sees

Caregiving is a kind of tired you have not been before. It is not just sleep deprivation, though there is plenty of that. It is a layered exhaustion.

- **Physical** — from the lifting, the driving, the running between appointments, the sleeping with one ear open.
- **Mental** — from holding the entire schedule in your head, the medications, the insurance status, the appointment changes, the names of the people you've talked to today.
- **Emotional** — from the constant low-grade fear, the grief that hasn't started but is already there, the hope that flickers and goes out and flickers again.
- **Decision fatigue** — from making, on average, dozens of small medical and logistical decisions a day, each of which has consequences you can't fully predict.

People will look at you and say, "You look tired." You will smile and nod. You will not have words for what tired actually means right now. That's normal.

Guilt: The Forever Companion

Guilt is going to be your roommate. Get used to it. It will show up in a hundred forms:

- Guilt for not being there enough.
- Guilt for being there so much that you've abandoned your own kids, your job, your marriage.
- Guilt for resenting your loved one when they're being demanding.
- Guilt for the moment of relief that flickered through you when you thought, "Once this is over, I can sleep."
- Guilt for snapping at the nurse.
- Guilt for not snapping at the nurse when she deserved it.

- Guilt for not visiting your siblings' kids this year.
- Guilt for missing a dose, a side effect, a question you should have asked, a sign you should have caught.

Some of this guilt is appropriate. Most of it is not. Guilt does not equal evidence of wrongdoing. Sometimes it is just the cost of caring about somebody.

Try this: when guilt shows up, name it out loud. "I'm feeling guilty for sleeping in this morning." Then ask yourself: "If my best friend told me she was feeling this, what would I tell her?" Whatever you'd say to her is true for you, too.

Anger: The Emotion People Don't Talk About

You are going to get angry. Not just inconvenienced. Furious. White-hot angry. At:

- Insurance companies.
- Doctors who didn't listen.
- Nurses who were cold.
- Family members who disappeared.
- Family members who showed up only to second-guess everything.
- Friends who asked once and never followed up.
- Your loved one, sometimes, for reasons you can't even fully name.
- Yourself, for not being able to do this gracefully.

Anger is not the opposite of love. It often runs underneath it. The mother you love is also the mother who is yelling at you for the third time today about something that isn't your fault. The husband you love is also the husband who is making decisions you think are stupid. You can love someone fully and be furious with them. Both are real.

The trick is not to suppress the anger — it leaks out somewhere bad if you do — but also not to discharge it onto the wrong target. Find a way to put it down for ten minutes. Take a walk around the building. Yell into a pillow. Text a trusted friend the unfiltered version. Then come back.

Grief That Starts Before the Loss

There is a real, named thing called **anticipatory grief.** It is the grief you feel before someone is gone, when you know they are going. It is the grief of watching someone you love change, decline, or disappear in pieces.

Anticipatory grief is real. It is not "getting ahead of yourself." It is not weakness. It is not pessimism. It is the human heart preparing itself for what it knows is coming.

It can hit at strange moments. Looking at an old photograph. Hearing them laugh in a way they used to laugh more often. Watching them sleep. Watching them not be able to do something they used to do without thinking.

Don't fight the anticipatory grief. Don't tell yourself you shouldn't be sad yet. Cry in the parking lot if you need to. Then go back in.

Feeling Like You're Failing (Even When You're Not)

Almost every caregiver I know feels like they are failing. Constantly. The bar they hold themselves to is impossible — the one where you respond to every text, manage every appointment perfectly, never miss a med, never lose patience, also keep your job, also raise your kids, also stay healthy, also be emotionally available to your spouse, also remember to send the birthday card.

Nobody can do all of that. You can't either. Not because you're insufficient — because what's being asked of you is more than one human can hold.

If you are feeding your loved one, getting them to their appointments, mostly remembering their meds, and asking questions when something's wrong — you are doing it. The version of you that exists in your head, the one who would handle all this perfectly, doesn't exist. The version of you that is showing up exhausted and scared and doing this anyway is the real one. That one is enough.

The Invisible Weight

Caregivers carry a lot of weight that nobody else can see.

- The mental load of every appointment, refill, follow-up, lab result.
- The constant low-level vigilance — always half-listening for a cough, a fall, a change.
- The anticipatory planning — "what if she falls tonight," "what if the labs are bad," "what if I can't take next Friday off."
- The performance — having to be cheerful in front of your loved one, professional in front of clinicians, calm on the phone with insurance, brave when you call your sister.
- The grief that has not started yet but is already taking up space.

This weight does not show up on your face most days. It does not show up on the family group chat. The people around you may genuinely have no idea how much you are holding. That is not their fault, and it is not yours either. But it does mean you have to consciously tell people. Otherwise nobody will know.

When the Weight Finally Cracked Through

I want to tell you about Thanksgiving 2023.

I think that was the first time I really started to admit to myself that I was depressed. Not just tired. Not just stressed. Depressed. From everything — the caregiving, the work, the mothering, and the constant knowledge that at any moment I was going to become a widow. Things had just gotten hard in a way that was different from the regular hard.

I was crying more. I was holding less. And I did the only thing I knew to do: I picked up the phone and called the office of the psychiatrist who worked within the health system where I worked, and I made an appointment.

I got the help I needed. We decided to try some medication. And in the process of figuring all of that out, I was diagnosed with ADHD — something that had gone unrecognized my entire life. Starting the medication helped more than I can put into words. But so did the therapist. Having someone whose entire job was to sit there and listen to me talk — and yes, sometimes just bitch — was a godsend.

I say all of this because I am a nurse. A healthcare administrator. Someone who has spent her career helping other people navigate exactly these systems. And I still needed help. I still almost waited too long to ask for it.

If you are reading this and something in this chapter is hitting too close — if the exhaustion has crossed into something darker, if the weight has stopped feeling manageable — please make the call. You don't have to have it all figured out before you call. You just have to call.

Loneliness in a Crowd

Caregiving is one of the loneliest jobs there is, even when you are surrounded by family. You are surrounded by people who love your loved one, but who don't know what you know. You are in rooms full of professionals who see your loved one as a chart, not a person. You are at parties where people ask, "How's your mom?" and they want a one-sentence answer, not the truth.

This loneliness is real. Pretending it isn't makes it worse. Things that help, even a little:

- **Find one person who can hear the unedited version.** A friend, a sibling, a therapist, a support group. Not someone who will fix it — someone who can sit with it.
- **Online caregiver communities.** Reddit, Facebook groups,

organizations specific to whatever your loved one has. The people there know the language. They've been in your kitchen at 2 a.m. too.

- **A therapist or counselor.** If you can swing it, do it. Many do sliding-scale. Some are covered by insurance. There is no medal for figuring this out alone.

If you're not sure where to start, call your primary care provider and ask for a referral. That's it. That's the whole first step. You don't have to have the right words. You just have to make the call. And if getting to an office feels impossible right now, online mental health services like BetterHelp make it easier to connect with a therapist from wherever you are — your car, your couch, your phone during a lunch break. The barrier to getting help has never been lower. Use that.

When the Relationship With Your Loved One Gets Hard

Caregiving changes the relationship. Sometimes for the better — there are tender moments you would not otherwise have had. But sometimes for the worse. The role reversal of becoming a parent's parent. The way illness can make a person more demanding, less appreciative, more frightened, more like a stranger.

Your loved one is also scared. They are losing autonomy. They are watching themselves change. They are angry, too, often at you, often unfairly, often because you are the safe person to be angry at.

This does not excuse cruelty. If your loved one is being verbally abusive, you are allowed to set a limit. "I love you, and I can't be yelled at like this. I'm going to step out for a few minutes." And then go.

It also doesn't excuse you when you snap. We all snap. The repair is what matters — "I was short with you earlier. I'm sorry. I love you." Said simply, then moved on. Repair, not perfection, is the work.

Letting In Help

Most caregivers are people who give. It is who you are. Asking feels like failing. It is not. It is the smartest thing you can do right now.

Most caregivers turn down help. They say "we're fine" when they are not fine. They believe they should be able to do it alone, or that asking is a burden, or that nobody will help correctly so why bother.

Try this instead. The next time someone says, "Let me know if you need anything," say one of these:

- "Thanks. Could you bring dinner Tuesday? I don't care what."
- "Yes — could you sit with Mom for an hour Saturday so I can take a walk?"
- "Would you mind making the calls to the lab to chase down those results?"
- "Can you come over and just be here for an hour while I cry without explaining why?"

People want to help. Most of the time, they don't because they don't know what would actually be useful. Tell them. They will rise.

I want to share what this looked like for me, because I think it matters.

In the last month of Dave's life I was able to stay home with him. And even though I had spent years being the person who did everything on her own, I finally relented. I let people help me.

The people I worked with at the time came together and brought us dinner five nights a week. It sounds simple. It was anything but. That one thing — not having to think about feeding us at the end of an exhausting day — took something significant off my plate at a time when my plate was overflowing. It was one of the most meaningful things anyone has ever done for me.

I didn't ask for it. They offered and I said yes. That was enough. Sometimes that's all it takes — just saying yes when someone offers.

Things That Help, Even a Little

- **Sleep, when you can get it.** Even a 30-minute nap matters.

- **Sunlight.** Step outside daily, even for five minutes.
- **Movement.** Walk around the block. Stretch. Anything.
- **Eating.** Cereal counts. Crackers count. Calories matter even when nothing tastes good.
- **Crying.** When you need to. It is a release valve, not a weakness.
- **Laughing.** Watch something stupid. Caregivers often forget that humor is allowed.
- **One thing that is just for you, every day.** A cup of coffee in silence. A song. A bath. A book. Five minutes is enough.
- **Getting professional help when you need it.** Not when it gets bad enough. Now. Before the Thanksgiving when you finally can't hold it anymore.

Things That Make It Worse

- **Drinking too much.** It feels like relief. It is mostly delay.
- **Comparing yourself to other caregivers.** They are also lying about how it's going.
- **Reading too many medical articles at 2 a.m.**
- **Doom-scrolling medical information and support groups at midnight.** There is a difference between being informed and feeding the fear. Know which one you're doing.
- **Trying to control the family members who aren't helping.** You can ask. You cannot make them. Save the energy.
- **Believing that being strong means not needing anything.**

When You Need More Than This Chapter Can Give

If you are experiencing thoughts of self-harm, persistent hopelessness, an inability to function, or a sense that you can't go on — please tell someone. Your own doctor. A therapist. The 988 Suicide and Crisis Lifeline. Caregiving is hard enough without doing it inside a depression that no one is treating.

There is no extra credit for suffering quietly. There is help. You are allowed to use it.

Do This Next

- **Tell one person, today, the truth about how you're doing.** Not the pleasantries. The actual truth. Pick someone safe.
- **Schedule something — anything — that is just for you in the next seven days.** Coffee with a friend. A walk. A movie alone. Put it on the calendar like an appointment.
- **If you've been white-knuckling this alone, find a therapist or a caregiver support group.** Even one session. Even one meeting.
- **Look into BetterHelp or ask your PCP for a referral** if getting to an office feels impossible. The first step is smaller than you think.
- **Try the script:** the next time someone says "let me know how I can help," say one specific thing. See what happens.
- **If something in this chapter hit too close — if you recognized yourself in the depression, the exhaustion, the weight that won't lift — make the call.** Today. Not when it gets worse. Today.

In the next chapter, we're going to go deeper into self-care — the realistic kind, not the glossy kind. The kind that fits inside actual caregiving life.

Chapter Fifteen

Taking Care of Yourself (Without Feeling Like an Asshole)

Self-Care That Fits Inside Actual Caregiving

Let me guess. You picked up a self-care book once. It told you to wake up at 5 a.m., journal for 30 minutes, drink lemon water, do yoga, take a long bath, and meditate. You laughed and put the book down. You then went back to figuring out whether the home health agency was supposed to come Tuesday or Wednesday.

Most self-care advice is written by people who have not been a caregiver.

The version that fits inside this life is different. It is smaller. It is grittier. It is less Instagram-able. And it actually works.

This chapter is about that version.

Why Self-Care Feels Impossible

It feels impossible because, mostly, it is. The life of a caregiver does not allow for an hour of yoga. There are not extra hours. The pretense that there are is part of why caregivers feel so guilty when they fail at "self-care."

Three real reasons self-care collapses for caregivers:

- **Time scarcity.** Every minute you spend on yourself is a minute you didn't spend on them.
- **Guilt.** "Mom is sick. How dare I take a bath."
- **Energy depletion.** Even when you have the time, you are too tired to use it.

Knowing this, the goal is not to become someone with a 90-minute morning routine. The goal is to find the smallest sustainable practices that keep you from collapsing. We're going to call that **bare minimum survival care.**

Bare Minimum Survival Care

Here is the floor. The non-negotiable, this-is-what-keeps-you-functional version. If you do nothing else, do these:

- **Eat something three times a day.** It does not have to be a meal. A protein bar counts. A handful of crackers and a glass of milk counts. Hunger turns into rage and bad decisions.
- **Drink water.** A bottle next to you, refilled. Dehydration produces fatigue and headaches you'll mistake for caregiver burnout.
- **Sleep when you can.** Six hours is better than four. Even a 20-minute nap. If you can't sleep at night, sleep when they sleep.
- **Move your body once a day for at least ten minutes.** Walking the parking lot. Stretching while the coffee makes. Up and down the stairs three times. The point is movement, not fitness.
- **Step outside daily, even briefly.** Sunlight regulates your

sleep, mood, and circadian rhythm in ways nothing else does.

- **Talk to one human you like, every day.** A text counts. A two-minute phone call counts. Isolation accelerates everything bad about caregiving.

That's the floor. If you can hit those six, you have the chance of staying functional. Anything beyond that is bonus.

Recharge Practices That Take Five Minutes or Less

Some realistic options for the moments when you have a tiny sliver of time.

- **Step outside.** Even into a parking lot. Look at the sky for two minutes.
- **Box breathing.** Inhale for 4, hold for 4, exhale for 4, hold for 4. Three rounds. Lowers heart rate, clears head.
- **Cold water on your face.** Sounds ridiculous. Resets the nervous system. Try it.
- **Music.** One song. Headphones. Whatever you would have danced to in college. Loud.
- **Text the friend who makes you laugh.** Don't apologize for not texting in a while. Just text.
- **Sit in your car for five minutes before going inside.** Don't apologize for this either. It's a real thing.
- **Stretch.** Ten arm circles, forward fold, neck rolls. Done in two minutes.
- **Pet an animal.** Real, measurable nervous system effects. Steal a dog if you have to.
- **Hum or sing something.** Anything. In the car, in the shower, doesn't matter.
- **Hold a warm cup of coffee or tea with both hands and just drink it.** No phone. No scrolling.
- **Light a candle.** Sit near it for two minutes.

- **Write three things down** — anything that's in your head. Get it out of there.
- **Put your feet on the floor, close your eyes, and just breathe for sixty seconds.**
- **Step away from the screen.** Any screen. For five minutes.
- **Wash your hands slowly.** Feel the water. Don't rush it.
- **Look out a window for two minutes.** Not at your phone. Out a window.
- **Do something creative for ten minutes.** Doodle. Color. Write three sentences. Make something with your hands. You don't have to be good at it.

What Mine Looked Like

I want to tell you what mine looked like, because it probably isn't what you'd expect.

When Dave was sick, my self-care was creative. I worked with resin — making art, mixing colors, watching something take shape under my hands. I wrote stories. I bought a laser engraver and taught myself how to use it. None of it was productive in the caregiving sense. None of it solved anything. But it gave my brain somewhere else to live for an hour, and that hour kept me sane.

I didn't call it self-care at the time. I called it something I needed to do. Turns out those are the same thing.

Your version doesn't have to look like anyone else's. It doesn't have to be expensive, Instagram-worthy, or even make sense to anyone outside your own head. It just has to be yours. Something that gives you back a version of yourself that isn't the caregiver. Hold onto that.

The Boundaries Conversation

Boundaries are how you make sure caregiving does not eat your entire life. They are not selfish. They are structural. People who have no boundaries don't last — they burn out, get sick, become resentful, or break. Boundaries are what keep you in the game long enough to actually be there.

With Family

This is where most boundary work needs to happen. Common situations:

- **The sibling who isn't pulling their weight.** "I need you to take Mom to the cardiologist next Wednesday. I can't do every appointment. If you can't, who can we ask?" Concrete ask, not a guilt trip.
- **The relative who criticizes from a distance.** "I'm doing my best. I'm not going to keep talking about whether I'm doing it right with someone who isn't here. If you'd like to help, I'd love that."
- **The family member who asks for updates constantly.** Set a routine. "I'll send a text update every Sunday night. If something major changes, I'll call. Otherwise, please don't text me daily — I can't keep up."
- **Your loved one's behavior, when it crosses lines.** "I love you. I cannot be talked to like this. I'm going to step out for a few minutes and come back when we can talk respectfully."

With Work

- **Talk to HR about FMLA.** Family Medical Leave Act protects your job for unpaid leave for caregiving. Twelve weeks of protected time per year (federal minimum).
- **Have an honest conversation with your manager.** Not over-sharing, but enough that they understand. Most people are more flexible than caregivers expect, but only if they know.
- **Use your PTO.** It's yours. You earned it. Don't save it for later.
- **If your job genuinely doesn't allow flexibility,** weigh whether the job is sustainable through this. Hard conversation, but real. And worth asking yourself — if they can't be flexible during one

of the hardest seasons of your life, is this really the place you want to work?

With Yourself

This is the hardest one. The boundary you set with yourself is what stops you from doing fourteen things when you should be doing three.

- **Some days, you are not going to make every call.** That is not failure. That is triage.
- **You don't have to be there for every appointment.** Sometimes the case manager or another family member can. Practice saying yes to that.
- **You are allowed to take a day off from caregiving.** Not symbolically — actually. A whole day. Once a month if you can manage it. The world does not collapse. (It feels like it will. It won't.)

The Bare Minimum Survival Day

On the worst days, this is the version. Print it, post it on the fridge, lower the bar that low when you need to.

- **Get dressed.** Pajamas off, real clothes on. Even sweatpants count if they're not the ones you slept in.
- **Eat three times.**
- **Drink water.**
- **Step outside once.** Five minutes.
- **Sleep tonight.** Whatever it takes — melatonin, an early bedtime, swapping the night shift with someone.
- **Talk to one safe person.** Two-minute call, a text, a wave at a neighbor.

That's it. If you got through one of those days, you didn't fail. You survived. Surviving is enough some days.

Asking for Help (Specifically)

We talked about this in the last chapter, but it bears repeating — and expanding. Because most caregivers need to hear it more than once.

People want to help. They are mostly bad at guessing what would help. Make a list. Keep it on your phone. The next time someone says "what can I do?" pull from it.

Sample Help-Wanted List

- Bring a meal.
- Sit with [my person] for an hour so I can sleep.
- Take [my person] to one appointment this month.
- Do my grocery run.
- Pick up the kids from school.
- Mow my lawn.
- Drop off coffee at the hospital.
- Call the insurance company about the claim from 3/14.
- Sit with me at chemo.
- Just text me randomly to check on me.

Match the size of the help to the relationship. Closer people get bigger asks. Acquaintances get small ones. People who said "I'd really like to help" twice get bigger ones than people who say it once at a party.

Therapy, Support Groups, and Professional Help

These are not failure. They are infrastructure.

- **Therapy.** A trained outside person who is not invested in any side of your family. Many therapists specialize in caregivers, grief, or chronic illness. Sliding scale exists. Online options like BetterHelp, Open Path, and Talkspace exist. I found mine through the health system I worked in. You can find yours through your PCP, your insurance portal, or Psychology Today's therapist finder at psychologytoday.com.

- **Caregiver support groups.** In-person through hospitals, hospices, faith communities. Online through Reddit (r/Caregiver-

Support, condition-specific subs), Facebook groups, organizations like the Family Caregiver Alliance.

- **EAP (Employee Assistance Program).** If your employer offers one, it usually includes a free chunk of counseling sessions. Use them.
- **Respite care.** Adult day programs, in-home respite hours, short overnight stays at a facility. Often covered by hospice, the VA, Medicaid waivers, or specific organizations. Ask the case manager what's available.

If You Are Drinking Too Much

Caregivers drink. It's normal, it's understandable, and it can quickly stop being okay. If you are drinking more than you used to, drinking earlier, drinking to fall asleep, or drinking to take the edge off your loved one's care — notice it. Notice it without judgment, but notice it.

Talk to your doctor or a therapist if it's tipped over. The earlier you address it, the easier. And it doesn't have to be alcohol. Self-medication is real — food, shopping, screens, substances of all kinds. Sometimes we don't even realize that's what we're doing until someone names it. Consider this it being named.

On Resentment

Resentment is a sign you have given more than you can sustain. It is not a moral failing. It is information.

If you are deeply resentful — of your loved one, of family who isn't helping, of friends, of the situation — something has to give. Either you take more, or you give less. The math has to balance.

Things you can change to give yourself more: more help (paid or unpaid), more boundaries, more honest conversations with family. Things you can't change: the diagnosis, the system, the relatives who will never step up.

Spend energy on what you can change. Save grief for what you can't.

Do This Next

- **Pick three of the bare minimum survival care items above. Today.** Write them on a sticky note. Stick it on the fridge.
- **Make the help-wanted list.** Save it on your phone.
- **One conversation, this week, where you set a boundary with someone.** Family member, work, your loved one. Practice the language out loud first.
- **Look at your calendar. Find one hour, in the next seven days, that is yours.** Block it. Protect it like an appointment.
- **Find your creative outlet.** Or remember the one you abandoned when caregiving started. Give it one hour this week. Not as a reward for finishing everything else. As a non-negotiable.
- **If you've been white-knuckling this without help, make one inquiry** — to a therapist, a support group, a respite program, an EAP. One call, one email.

This chapter is the one to come back to. The hardest part is not figuring out what works — it's giving yourself permission to do it. Do it anyway.

Up next: the chapter we don't want to write but have to. When the situation shifts — when treatment stops working, when conversations turn toward comfort instead of cure. The terminal chapter.

Chapter Sixteen

When It's Terminal (And No One Says It Out Loud)

The Hardest Conversation. The One That Matters Most.

There is a moment in many caregiving journeys when the energy in the room shifts and nobody quite acknowledges it.

Maybe the doctor has stopped talking about cures and started talking about "managing symptoms." Maybe a treatment is being recommended that isn't expected to extend life much, but is presented as if it might. Maybe your loved one is sleeping more, eating less, fading in ways you've started to feel but don't have the words for. Maybe you've been told something is "end stage," but no one has said the next word out loud.

This chapter is about that moment. About recognizing it. About what to ask. About what's available. About how to talk to your loved one about something neither of you wants to talk about. And about how to do all of this without rushing it, and without missing it.

This is the chapter I wish someone had handed me a long time before I needed it.

Recognizing the Shift

Healthcare often will not say the word "dying." Sometimes for legal reasons. Sometimes because the team isn't sure. Sometimes because they're trying to protect you, or themselves. So you have to read the signals.

Signs the conversation is shifting:

- **The treatment goals change.** "Cure" becomes "control." "Control" becomes "comfort." Listen for that drift.
- **The conversations get vaguer.** "We're hopeful but the prognosis is guarded." "It's hard to predict." "We should focus on quality of life." Each of those phrases is often code.
- **Treatments are being de-escalated.** Stopping chemo. Stopping aggressive antibiotics. Stopping dialysis. Stopping anything they were pushing hard six months ago.
- **Hospice is mentioned, even casually.** Sometimes a doctor will float the word and watch your reaction. Take it seriously. And please — do not treat hospice like He Who Must Not Be Named. It is a word. It is a resource. Say it out loud. We'll talk about it more in a minute.
- **Your loved one is getting smaller.** Eating less. Sleeping more. Pulling away. Talking less. Withdrawing from things they cared about.
- **Your gut keeps telling you something has changed.** It usually has.

If the team isn't naming it and you suspect it's there, you can name it. You are allowed to ask the question directly: **"Are we at a point**

where we should be thinking about hospice or comfort care?" That sentence shifts the whole room. It is okay to say it.

The Questions That Cut Through

If you want clarity, these specific questions tend to get past the vague answers.

- **"What is your best guess about how much time we have, in terms of months, weeks, or days?"** Doctors are notoriously bad at exact predictions, but most can give a range. Asking explicitly forces a real answer.
- **"If this were your mother, what would you do?"** Watch their face. The honest doctors will tell you. The honest ones often have a strong opinion they're not volunteering.
- **"What would you NOT do at this point?"** This is the question that catches the over-treatment we sometimes drift into. "At this point, I wouldn't push another round of chemo." "I wouldn't transfer her to ICU." That's information.
- **"What does the next month look like, if we keep treating? What does it look like if we transition to comfort?"** Side by side. Specific.
- **"What are the things that would make you tell us it's time for hospice?"** Sometimes named criteria help everyone get on the same page.
- **"What will the dying process look like for this disease?"** Hard question. Useful. Knowing what to expect prevents panic when it happens.

One thing worth knowing before you ask these questions: most doctors today are reluctant to give a specific timeline. Questions like "how long does he have?" are often met with answers like the one we received — "We don't want to put an expiration date on anyone."

And honestly? That's not a dodge. There's real truth behind it.

Research has shown that when people are given a specific expected timeframe, they often don't make it to that date. But when people aren't anchored to a number, they frequently surpass what anyone suspected. The mind and the body are connected in ways medicine still doesn't fully understand.

So when you ask these questions and the doctor gives you a range instead of a date, or talks about "weeks to months" instead of a specific number — that's not evasion. That's wisdom. Push for enough information to make good decisions. Don't push for a date that may do more harm than good.

Hospice vs Aggressive Treatment

There is a real choice here, and most families don't fully understand it. Let me lay it out.

Aggressive (Curative) Treatment

Continued chemotherapy, dialysis, surgeries, ICU-level interventions, ventilators, feeding tubes, aggressive antibiotic courses. The goal is to extend life or cure disease. The trade-off: side effects, hospital time, procedures, often a worse quality of life and sometimes a worse death.

Aggressive treatment can be the right choice — for someone with curable disease, for someone who values length over quality, for someone who's still mostly themselves and wants to keep fighting.

Aggressive treatment is sometimes the wrong choice when it's pursued because nobody had the conversation. When the next round of chemo is started not because there's a real chance of benefit, but because nobody named the alternative. When the ventilator goes in because it's 2 a.m. in the ER and no one had asked, ahead of time, what the patient actually wanted.

There is also a middle path many families never hear about: continuing some treatments for comfort or function while stopping others.

Radiation to shrink a painful tumor, even when cure isn't the goal. Antibiotics for an infection that's causing suffering, even in hospice. The lines are not always as hard as they seem. Ask the palliative care team what's possible.

Hospice

Hospice is care focused on comfort instead of cure, for people whose physicians estimate they have six months or less if the disease runs its course. It is covered by Medicare, Medicaid, and most insurance, often at 100%. It is one of the most comprehensive benefits in healthcare, and it is wildly underused.

Hospice usually includes:

- A nurse who visits regularly (often weekly) and is on call 24/7.
- A home health aide for help with bathing, hygiene, light personal care.
- A social worker.
- A chaplain (you can decline if you want).
- Volunteers.
- Medications related to the terminal diagnosis, delivered to the home.
- Equipment — hospital bed, oxygen, commode, anything needed for comfort.
- Bereavement support for the family for up to 13 months after death.

Hospice can happen at home, in a hospice house, or in a nursing facility. It is not a place — it is a service. The team comes to wherever the patient is.

The biggest myth: "Hospice means giving up." It does not. It means changing the goal from cure to comfort. People can come off hospice if their condition unexpectedly improves. People can choose to go back to hospital-level care. Hospice is a service, not a one-way door.

The second biggest myth: "It's too soon for hospice." Most families enroll too late. The average length of hospice service in the US is shorter than people imagine — sometimes only days. Earlier hospice means more support, more comfort, and often a better death. Better for the patient. Better for you.

If you're wondering whether hospice could be appropriate, ask. The intake is usually free and informational. Asking does not commit you to anything.

How Hospice Came Into Our Lives

I want to tell you how hospice came into our lives, because I think it matters.

For a long time, hospice was treated like a dirty word in our house. Worse than a dirty word, honestly. Dave wasn't ready to give up, and bringing up hospice felt like suggesting he should. So we didn't.

In November 2024, we learned that his renal cell cancer was spreading further into his abdomen. There was even a scare that it was blocking his colon. He wasn't actively dying — not in the way you picture it. But something shifted in me.

I brought up hospice. And I'll be honest with you: I did it selfishly.

I explained it to Dave exactly that way. I told him I wanted to get established with a hospice team now — not because I thought he was going to die next month, not because I was giving up on him, but because I wanted the resource in place for when we needed it. I told him that being on hospice didn't mean he had to stop fighting. It just meant that when he decided enough was enough, we would already have a team ready. We wouldn't be starting from scratch in the hardest moment.

He agreed. And I was so glad he did.

When April 2025 came, I was so grateful we had already done

this. One phone call. That was all it took. They were there — with everything we needed, everything I needed — because the relationship was already built. The paperwork was done. The team knew us. We didn't have to figure any of it out in the worst days of our lives.

If you are reading this and hospice feels like a dirty word — I understand. I lived that. But I want you to hear what I told Dave: getting established doesn't mean giving up. It means being ready. And being ready, when the time comes, is one of the greatest gifts you can give the person you love.

Palliative Care vs Hospice

These are different and the words get confused.

- **Palliative care** is comfort-focused care that can be added to active treatment at any stage of a serious illness. You can have chemo and palliative care. You can have dialysis and palliative care. The goal is to manage symptoms, regardless of treatment status.
- **Hospice** is a specific type of palliative care, intended for the end of life, with the active treatment for the terminal diagnosis stopped.

Many people benefit from palliative care for years before they ever consider hospice. If your loved one has serious illness and significant symptoms, ask: "Would palliative care be appropriate now?"

Palliative care is typically available through a referral from your provider. It can be delivered in the hospital, in a clinic, or sometimes at home. If your loved one's provider hasn't mentioned it and symptoms are significant, ask directly: "Can we get a palliative care referral?" You don't have to wait to be offered it.

Hard Conversations With Your Loved One

Here is something I want to say before we go any further: these conversations shouldn't wait until someone is sick. Have them now. Have them with everyone you love, while everyone is healthy and there's no urgency and no one is scared.

I knew for years that Dave wanted to be cremated. That was never a question. Where we had some disagreement was on his service. I remember the conversation — he told me he didn't want a funeral, just cremation. No service.

I'll be honest with you. I told him that at that point, it wouldn't matter what he wanted. He'd be dead. The funeral wasn't for him. It was for me, and his mother, and everyone else who loved him — so we could have somewhere to put our grief and some closure to hold onto.

He didn't argue.

The point is: have the conversation. Have it early. Have it when it's almost a little funny, when you can push back on each other and laugh about it. Because when the time actually comes, you want to already know. And the people who love them need what they need too — and that is just as valid.

Most people, when offered the chance, will tell you what they want — if you ask, and if they trust you to handle the answer.

Ways to start the conversation:

"I know we don't usually talk about this, and we don't have to right now. But I want to make sure that if something happens — something we don't want — I'm able to make decisions the way you would want them made. Can we talk about what matters to you?"

"The doctor said something today that scared me a little. I want to ask you what you'd want if it ever came to that."

"If you could choose, what would matter most to you in how this goes?"

Then listen. Don't argue. Don't talk them out of it. Don't change the subject. Their answer might surprise you.

Some people won't want to have this conversation. They'll change the subject, deflect, or get angry. That's okay. Plant the seed. Come back another day. Try a different door. Some people need to hear the question more than once before they're ready to answer it. And some people will never be ready — and you'll have to make decisions with the information you have. That's okay too.

Specific questions to walk through, when the moment is right:

- Where do you want to be, at the end? Home? Hospital? Hospice house? Nursing facility?
- Are there things you do not want? Tube feedings? Ventilator? CPR? Aggressive interventions?
- Are there things you do want? Pain controlled? Family present? Music? Specific people there or not there?
- Do you want to die at home if at all possible?
- Who do you want making decisions if you can't?

These conversations are not one-and-done. They evolve. Have them more than once. Things change.

Advance Directives, POLST, and Code Status

Paper exists to make wishes enforceable. The basics:

- **Living will.** A document expressing what kinds of care you want or don't want at the end of life. Specific to circumstances — for example, whether you want to be kept on a ventilator if you can't breathe on your own, or whether you want a feeding tube if you can no longer eat.
- **Healthcare power of attorney (HCPOA) — also called a Medical Power of Attorney (MPOA).** These are the same thing, just named differently depending on where you live. This document names the person who can make medical decisions for the patient if they can't make them for themselves. It is important to understand that this only covers healthcare-related decisions — it has no authority over finances, property, bank accounts, or other assets. If you need someone to manage financial matters, that requires a separate and different type of power of attorney entirely. For anything involving

finances, assets, or estate planning, please consult an attorney or estate planning professional. That conversation is worth having at the same time you're handling the medical paperwork — while everyone is healthy and clear-headed enough to make good decisions.

- **Advance directive.** Often refers to the combination of a living will and a healthcare power of attorney in a single document. Different states have different forms — your hospital, your doctor's office, or your state health department website can provide the correct one for where you live.
- **POLST / MOLST / POST.** These stand for Physician Orders for Life-Sustaining Treatment, Medical Orders for Life-Sustaining Treatment, and Physician Orders for Scope of Treatment — the name varies by state, but the purpose is the same. It's a medical order signed by a physician that translates a person's wishes into actionable instructions that paramedics, hospitals, and facilities are required to follow. Critical for people with serious illness who want to avoid certain interventions.
- **DNR / DNI.** Do Not Resuscitate and Do Not Intubate. Specific orders that tell medical teams not to perform CPR or place a breathing tube if the patient stops breathing or their heart stops. Without these orders in place, the default is full code — meaning paramedics and hospital staff will do everything possible, including chest compressions, electric shocks to the heart, and ventilator placement. If your loved one wouldn't want that, the order has to be in place, signed, and visible.

Get these done before you need them. It is much, much easier to set up paperwork during a calm afternoon than during a 2 a.m. ER visit.

Once you have these documents, make sure the right people have copies. The primary care provider. The specialist. The hospital if your loved one has been admitted recently. The facility if they're in one. A copy at home in a visible place — not locked in a drawer, not in a safe deposit box at the bank. First responders cannot wait for you to find the paperwork. It needs to be findable in thirty seconds.

What Dying Often Actually Looks Like

If you've never been with someone at the end, you may not know what to expect. The clinical version, in plain English, helps.

- **Eating and drinking decrease.** This is not starvation — it's the body shutting down. Forcing food can cause distress. Small sips of water, ice chips, swabs for the mouth are all comfort measures.
- **Sleeping increases.** A lot. People often sleep most of the last days. They are still aware sometimes — keep talking gently, even when they don't respond.
- **Breathing changes.** Sometimes irregular, sometimes shallow, sometimes with longer pauses. "Cheyne-Stokes" breathing — cycles of fast then slow then pauses — is common in the final hours.
- **Terminal secretions (sometimes called the death rattle).** A gurgling sound from secretions in the throat the person can no longer clear. It often distresses families more than the patient. Hospice nurses can help manage it with positioning and medication.
- **Cool, mottled extremities.** Hands and feet may turn blue or purple in the last day or two as circulation pulls inward.
- **Restlessness or agitation.** Common. Hospice can help with medications.
- **The actual moment is often very quiet.** Many families describe it as gentler than they feared.

Many people die in the few minutes when their family steps out — to get coffee, to use the bathroom, to take a call. Some hospice nurses believe people choose this. That they wait for a moment alone. If you weren't there at the exact moment, please hear this: you were there. You showed up, every day. The moment of death is one minute of many thousands. Don't let that one minute erase all the others.

If you don't want to read this section, skip it. If you want to read it now and not in the moment, this is when. Knowing helps.

The Family Around You

End-of-life situations bring out the best and worst in families. Old wounds open. Siblings revert to childhood roles. Strong opinions emerge from people who have been absent.

A few things that help:

- **A family meeting with the medical team** to make sure everyone hears the same information.
- **A clear decision-maker** (the named healthcare power of attorney). One person, not three.
- **Permission to disagree without it derailing care.** Family members may grieve differently and want different things. The patient's wishes — not majority vote — lead.
- **A social worker or hospice chaplain** can sometimes help mediate.

And then there is the family member who has been absent through all of it — the appointments, the hospital stays, the hard days — who suddenly appears at the end with opinions and demands. This is incredibly common and incredibly painful. You don't have to give them equal authority. The healthcare power of attorney is the decision-maker. The people who showed up are the ones who know what's been happening. If someone wants to be part of the last chapter, they don't get to rewrite the ones they missed.

Saying Goodbye

There is no script for this. There also isn't a wrong way.

Some people want big conversations. Some want small ones — a hand squeeze, a movie watched together, dinner that nobody named as the last dinner.

Some things people often want to say, given the chance: "I love you." "Thank you." "I forgive you." "Please forgive me." "It's okay." "You can let go."

Say what is yours to say. Don't wait until the last hour. The last hour, sometimes, isn't the moment they hear best.

And if your loved one is still well — if this chapter feels premature for where you are right now — say the things anyway. "I love you." "Thank you." "I'm glad you're mine." Don't save them for the end. The end is not a guaranteed conversation.

Do This Next

- **If your loved one is seriously ill and the conversation has not happened, start it.** This week. Not tomorrow. "I want to make sure I know what you would want" — that's the whole opening.
- **Find out if hospice or palliative care could be appropriate now.** Ask the doctor directly. Ask the case manager. Ask without committing to anything.
- **Get the paperwork done.** Healthcare power of attorney. Advance directive. POLST if appropriate. The kitchen table is the right place for this. Not the ICU.
- **Make sure documents are findable.** Not in a drawer. Not in a safe. Somewhere a first responder can find in thirty seconds.
- **If you are facing this right now,** find a hospice nurse or palliative care provider. They are some of the most competent, compassionate people in healthcare. They will help you through the parts you can't see yet.
- **Tell someone how you're doing.** This is the chapter that breaks the most caregivers. Don't carry it alone.

Up next: the chapter that comes after. After the loss. What happens when the caregiving ends, and life keeps going.

Chapter Seventeen

After It's Over

The Quiet After. The Paperwork. The Grief That Doesn't Follow a Schedule.

There is a moment after a death — sometimes hours, sometimes a day — when the house gets quiet and you don't know what to do next. The pumps and the alarms have stopped. The hospice team has come and gone. The body has been taken. The phone calls have started. And you are standing in the kitchen at a strange time of day, holding a coffee mug, with no one to give a medication to.

It is the quietest your house has been in months. Maybe years.

This chapter is about what comes next. The practical things you have to handle. And the fact that grief does not follow a schedule, and you are not failing if it does not look the way you thought it would.

The First 48 Hours

Right after a death, a lot of small things have to happen. You don't have to do them perfectly. You just have to do them.

- **If your loved one was on hospice, call hospice first** — even if the hospice nurse isn't physically present. As long as hospice is involved in the care, they handle the pronouncement and coordinate with the funeral home. That's what they're there for.

- **If your loved one was not on hospice and dies at home, call 911.** Law enforcement will respond — this is routine, not an investigation. A medical examiner will also be involved, and depending on the circumstances, they will determine whether your loved one goes to the medical examiner's office first or directly to the funeral home. This process can feel alarming if you don't know it's coming. It is standard. Let it happen.
- **Notify close family.** Whatever order makes sense to you. There is no right way.
- **Funeral home arrangements.** Most families have a funeral home in mind, even if loosely. The funeral home will pick up the body and coordinate with the hospice team or with you directly.
- **Decisions about cremation, burial, services.** Some of this can wait a day. Some — if there's a specific cultural or religious timeframe — cannot. Make the decisions you have to. Defer the rest.
- **Death certificate.** The funeral home usually orders these for you. Order more copies than you think you'll need. Ten is not too many. You will need certified copies for banks, insurance, Social Security, retirement accounts, the deed, the car title, and more. Some funeral homes can order extra copies for a small fee — but your local courthouse may be able to provide those same certified copies for free. It's worth checking before you pay.

The Phone Calls and the Notifications

Over the next few days and weeks, a lot of organizations need to be notified. You don't have to do them all in one day.

In the First Week

- **Funeral home** — services, transport, paperwork.
- **Social Security Administration** — to stop benefits and report the death. The funeral home often does this on your behalf, but verify. In some cases the state notifies them automatically — we

received a letter from Social Security on the day of Dave's funeral letting us know they were already aware. But don't assume. Notify them anyway. Survivors may also be eligible for benefits — ask.

- **Pension provider, retirement accounts** — stop ongoing payments and ask about survivor benefits.
- **Health insurance** — stop the policy.
- **Life insurance company** — you can contact them right away, but they cannot process any claims until a certified death certificate is in hand. This is why having plenty of copies matters.
- **Employer (if working at time of death)** — for final pay, benefits, and HR paperwork.

In the First Month

- **Banks and financial institutions.** Make sure your name is on accounts wherever possible — before this moment. When Dave passed on a Friday, his debit card was disconnected by Monday because the bank had already learned of his passing. Thankfully my name was on the account, or I would not have been able to access the funds.
- Credit card companies.
- Mortgage or landlord.
- Utilities (if transferring).
- Vehicle titles.
- Voter registration.
- Passport cancellation.
- **Subscriptions and recurring charges.** Check bank and credit card statements carefully — recurring charges often reveal accounts you didn't know existed. Cancel what needs canceling.
- **Digital accounts** — email, social media, online banking, streaming services, cloud storage. Some platforms have a legacy contact or memorialization process. Others require a death certificate and legal documentation to close.

The best advice I can give you: if at all possible, get all of this in order before your loved one passes. Make sure accounts are accessible. Know where the documents are. Know who the executor of the estate is and make sure they understand that responsibility. The governmental red tape after a death is not a simple process. Someone has to carry it — and doing even a little preparation ahead of time will save enormous time and heartache when the moment comes.

Organizing the Paperwork

Three things that keep this manageable:

- **A folder or binder for death certificates and all correspondence.** Everything in one place.
- **A simple log of what's been done.** "4/22 — notified Social Security. 4/24 — submitted life insurance claim. 4/26 — met with funeral home for final bill." The log keeps you sane when something asks "did I already do this?"
- **A trusted person to help.** Even if it's just to sit with you while you make a phone call.

A Note on Advance Directives After the Death

If your loved one had advance directives, a POLST, or a DNR on file — notify the relevant providers that these are no longer needed and can be removed from active records. The hospice team or primary care provider can help with this. Hold onto your own copies for your records.

Money Realities You Should Know

- **You are not personally responsible for most of your loved one's debts** unless you co-signed. Don't let collection agencies tell you otherwise. Their debts are paid from the estate, if there's anything in it. If the estate is empty, most debts die.
- **Medical bills will keep arriving after your loved one passes** — sometimes for months. Apply the same rules from Chap-

ter 12. You are not automatically responsible for these either. Bills go through the estate. If the estate has no assets, most medical debt dies with the person. Don't pay anything under pressure before you understand what you actually legally owe. When in doubt, consult an estate attorney — many offer a free initial consultation.

- **Credit card companies are sometimes aggressive.** Ignore the pressure. Send a copy of the death certificate. They are required to back off.
- **Funeral costs are often the most immediate expense.** Most funeral homes will work with you on payment. Some life insurance proceeds can be assigned directly to the funeral home to expedite this.
- **Social Security has a small lump-sum death benefit** ($255 as of recent years) — the funeral home or surviving spouse can apply for it.
- **If your loved one was a veteran,** there are burial benefits, survivor benefits, and sometimes a veteran's cemetery available. Contact the VA — you may be entitled to more than you realize.

The Emotional Aftermath

After the death, expect:

- **Numbness.** Sometimes for days. Sometimes for weeks. This is normal.
- **Strange relief.** That you can sleep. That the calendar is empty. That the phone stopped ringing. The relief does not mean you didn't love them. It means caregiving was hard, and now it's over. Both can be true.
- **Guilt about the relief.** Also normal. Don't feed it.
- **Sadness in waves.** Not a tidy stages-of-grief progression. More like an ocean. Sometimes calm. Sometimes a wave catches you in the cereal aisle and you can't breathe.
- **Anger.** At the disease. At the system. At God if you believe. At

your loved one for leaving. At yourself for things you didn't do or said.

- **Identity loss.** "I was a caregiver. Now what am I?" This is real. You spent so much time being for them that you may have forgotten who you are without that role.
- **Physical symptoms.** Exhaustion that doesn't lift. Sleep disruption. Appetite changes. Hair loss. Aches. Grief lives in the body.
- **Strange nostalgia for the caregiving days.** Even the hard ones. Because you were close to them in a way you may never be close to anyone again.

All of these are within the range of normal. Grief does not follow a script. It also doesn't end on a schedule — "you should be over it by now" is something only people who haven't grieved say.

What the Weeks After Looked Like for Me

Let me tell you what the weeks after looked like for me.

The days immediately following were a blur of people and food and logistics. What was I going to wear to the funeral? What was Finnegan going to wear? What was Dave going to wear? There is a surreal quality to those decisions — choosing an outfit for someone who is no longer there to have an opinion about it.

The day after the funeral I went and bought a new couch. I couldn't stand looking at the spot on the old one where Dave had spent the last month of his life — unable to really talk, fading in ways I couldn't fully reach. I didn't know what was going on in his head in those last weeks. I still don't. The couch had to go.

In the weeks that followed I did all the things he had told me no to, for whatever reason. I painted the front porch black. I decided to go back to school and get my MBA. Small rebellions. Small reclamations.

Then came the estate. Then our wedding anniversary — not even two months later. We would have been married sixteen years that day. I couldn't handle the silence, so I made a dinner I actually liked, and then invited myself — and the food — over to my brother-in-law's house. Because some days you just can't be alone with it.

Things were different. They always would be.

It wasn't until October or November that I finally had enough of the bedroom and rearranged it. That felt like something. A small turning.

They say the second year is the hardest. I'll let you know in 355 days.

When Grief Becomes Something More

Most grief, even when it lasts a long time, is moving. Slowly, unpredictably, but moving. The frequency and intensity of the worst waves usually eases over months and years. Other days come in. You laugh. You go a whole afternoon without thinking about them, and then feel guilty for that, and then keep going.

Sometimes grief gets stuck. The clinical name is **prolonged grief disorder** or **complicated grief.** Signs:

- Months in, you are not able to function in basic ways.
- You cannot accept the death — it still feels surreal long after the funeral.
- You are intensely longing in a way that is not easing.
- You feel that life has no meaning, or that you don't want to be here.
- You are isolating, drinking too much, unable to sleep, unable to eat.

If any of these describe you several months in, please see a therapist or a doctor. Grief therapy is a real, effective specialty. Sometimes a brief course of treatment opens up the rest of your life. There is no virtue in suffering alone.

The Caregiver's Specific Grief

Caregivers grieve differently than other family members. You did the heavy lifting for years or months. You saw things others didn't.

You also lost the role that organized your daily life. You may grieve:

- **The person you lost,** of course.
- **The relationship you had,** including the version of it that existed before the illness.
- **Your own time,** the years you gave to caregiving.
- **The version of yourself** you used to be before this began.
- **The things you didn't get to do** because you were caregiving.
- **The friendships** that didn't survive your unavailability.
- **The career steps you didn't take,** the trips you didn't go on, the kids' games you missed.

All of these losses are real. Naming them helps.

Rebuilding

People will tell you to "get back to normal." There is no back. There is forward. A new normal, slowly built. Things that help:

- **Reclaim small parts of your life.** Restart a hobby. Reach out to a friend. Walk a route you used to walk.
- **Don't make huge decisions for the first year if you don't have to.** Selling the house, moving cities, major financial changes — grief impairs judgment in ways you can't always feel from the inside. Small reclamations are different. Painting the porch. Going back to school. Those are you coming back to yourself. That's allowed.
- **Honor them in small, sustainable ways.** A photo on the desk. A donation. A walk on their birthday.
- **Find people who knew them.** Talking about them keeps them present in a healthy way.
- **Find people who didn't know them.** New friendships, new spaces, where you can be more than the version of you who was caring for someone sick.
- **Be patient with yourself.** This is one of the great challenges of being human. You don't graduate from it. You learn to live with it.

If You Were the Primary Caregiver

You may need a check-up of your own. Caregiving takes a toll. Things to do for yourself in the months after:

- **See your own doctor.** Catch up on screenings, labs, anything you've been putting off.
- **See a therapist if you can.** Even a brief course.
- **Sleep.** A lot. Not productive, glamorous sleep. Real, deep recovery sleep.
- **Eat real food again.** The freezer of casseroles is fine, but eventually go to the store.
- **Move.** Walking, gentle exercise. Don't expect to bounce. Expect to slowly come back into your body.
- **Reconnect with people.** Slowly. They missed you.
- **Don't fill the empty time too fast.** The instinct is to throw yourself into work or a project. Let some empty be empty for a while.

You may find, when you finally slow down enough to take care of yourself, that things come up that had been hiding under the noise of caregiving. Physical things. Mental health things. That's not bad news — it's your body finally having space to tell you what it needs. Listen.

On What Was Worth It

There will come a moment when you look back on the caregiving years and see them differently than you saw them at the time. The exhaustion fades. The hard days don't disappear, but they sit alongside other things. The conversations you had. The moments you held a hand. The laughter at the most inappropriate times. The way you became a person you didn't know you could be.

Caregiving costs a lot. It also gives a lot, in ways that are not visible until later. You can grieve the cost and notice the gift. They are not at war.

Do This Next

- **If you are in the immediate aftermath,** do not try to do it all at once. Make a list. Do the next thing. Sleep when you can.
- **Order extra death certificates** — ten copies if you can swing it. Save yourself the future call.
- **Check bank and credit card statements** for recurring charges on accounts you may not know about. Cancel what needs canceling.
- **Pick one person to be your call buddy** for the paperwork days. Someone you can call after a hard one and just talk for ten minutes.
- **Don't make any major life decisions in the first year if you can avoid it.**
- **See your own doctor,** when you have the energy. You matter, too.
- **Find a grief resource that fits.** A therapist, a support group, a book, a walk in the woods. Whatever lets you feel without performing.
- **If you are the executor of the estate,** find an estate attorney or ask your local courthouse about resources. You don't have to figure out the legal process alone. And if you can get things in order before your loved one passes — do it. Future you will be grateful.
- **Notify relevant providers** that advance directives, POLSTs, or DNRs on file are no longer needed and can be removed from active records.

There is one chapter left. It's the one I would have wanted to read on day one, if any of us could read forward in time. It's everything I wish someone had told me at the beginning.

Take a breath. Meet me there.

Chapter Eighteen

What I Wish I Knew From the Beginning

If I Could Hand You a Letter on Day One, This Would Be It

If I could go back to the version of me who was just becoming a caregiver — the one who didn't yet know how big this was going to get — there are things I would say. Things I would underline. Things I would say twice.

This chapter is that letter. Some of it is practical. Some of it is emotional. All of it is what I wish someone had handed me at the start.

Lessons I Learned the Hard Way

1. Get Organized Before You Need To

The chaos of disorganization is a separate kind of suffering, layered on top of the actual hard parts. The notebook, the medication list, the photos of insurance cards — set them up before you need them, not in the middle of the ER. Half the panic of caregiving is information panic. Eliminate it early.

2. The System Is Not Designed For You

It was not built around you and your loved one. It was built around billing codes, productivity metrics, and risk management. Once I stopped expecting it to be intuitive, things got easier. The system isn't broken — it's working as designed. Your job is not to fix it. Your job is to navigate it.

3. Ask the Question Out Loud

So many of the worst caregiver moments come from a question that didn't get asked. "Is this the right dose?" "Is this normal?" "Are we treating this aggressively or for comfort?" "Is hospice a possibility?" The questions feel awkward. They feel pushy. They feel like asking out loud will somehow make the answer worse. It doesn't. Ask anyway.

4. Document Everything

Names, dates, times, what was said. Doesn't have to be fancy. A spiral notebook works. The single best habit I built during caregiving was writing down the name of every person I spoke to. It saved me three or four times when stories didn't match later.

5. The Bedside Nurse Is Your Best Friend

In a hospital, the bedside nurse is closer to the situation than anyone else, including the doctors. Be kind. Bring coffee. Ask their name. Thank them. They will tell you things you would not have learned otherwise.

6. Call the Pharmacist

Pharmacists are wildly underused. They know drugs in a way most doctors don't. If you have a med question — dose, interaction, side effect — the pharmacist will often answer faster and more completely than the prescriber's office. They don't charge for the call.

7. Don't Pay the First Bill

Wait for the EOB. Compare. Medical bills can have errors. Most can be reduced. None are urgent enough to pay before you've actually understood what they are.

8. A Denial Is Not the Final Answer

It is the start of a conversation, not the end of it. They say no hoping you'll go away. Most families do. The ones who push back usually win.

9. The Case Manager Is the Most Underused Resource in Healthcare

In a hospital, ask for the case manager on day one. They can move things doctors can't. They are the bridge between the medical world and the practical world (home health, equipment, rehab, insurance authorizations). Get the name. Get the number. Use them.

10. Hospice Is Not Giving Up

It is changing the goal. From cure to comfort. It is also one of the most comprehensive benefits in healthcare and is wildly underused. Most families who enroll wish they had enrolled sooner. If hospice has been mentioned, even once, take it seriously.

If your loved one has a terminal illness, start the conversation now. Even if it's just to connect through palliative care. Some hospices don't make you jump in all the way — there are bridge programs that ease you in. Think of it as the decaf version. You get the support without the full commitment yet.

11. The Conversation You're Avoiding Is the One That Matters

The hard conversation about what your loved one wants at the end — the one you've been waiting for the right moment to have — there is no right moment. Have it when it occurs to you that you should. The kitchen table is the right place. Not the ICU at 2 a.m.

12. Self-Care Isn't a Luxury

Think about the airplane safety briefing. They tell you to put your own oxygen mask on first — not because you matter more than anyone else, but because you can't help anyone if you've passed out.

Caregiving is the same. If you break, get sick, or fall apart from running yourself into the ground, who is going to be there for your loved one?

Self-care is the maintenance of the engine that is doing the caregiving. Eat. Drink. Sleep. Move. Step outside. Talk to one human a day. Not because you deserve it (you do, but that's not the argument). Because if you fall apart, the whole thing falls apart.

13. Your Family Will Surprise You. Both Ways.

Some people will rise to a level you didn't expect. Some will disappear. The ones you thought would help, sometimes don't. The ones you wrote off, sometimes do the most.

Some will get mean and pushy. Remember — that's their emotions running the show. It can feel like it's about you, but it's not. It's about them. Keep doing what you're doing. Keep your head up. You are the one caring for your loved one. They are the ones being loud.

Try not to settle scores during the caregiving years — you will need clarity later. But also, take notes. The patterns you see now will inform how you spend your energy going forward.

14. You Will Make Mistakes

You will miss a sign. You will forget a med. You will skip an appointment. You will lose your temper. You will say something you wish you hadn't. None of this means you are failing at caregiving. It means you are a human doing an inhuman job. Forgive yourself. Repair when you can. Move on.

15. The Time Is Worth It

The hours, the conversations, the small moments, the bad days, the harder days. Even the parts that felt like loss as you were living them. The time you spent close to someone you love, when they needed you, will not feel wasted. Whatever else it was, it was that. Hold onto that part.

Mistakes I Made

In the spirit of being honest — things I got wrong, so you don't have to.

- **I tried to do everything alone.** It cost me sleep, friendships, and at least one bad decision I could have avoided if I'd let someone else carry a piece.
- **I let exhaustion erode my judgment.** I made decisions I would have made differently with eight hours of sleep.
- **I postponed my own grief until 'after.'** It came anyway, in the middle, in the wrong moments, harder because I'd been holding it back.
- **I put work above too many other things.** I kept telling myself I needed a steady job for when Dave was gone. I did need an income — but I didn't need it like that. Some of those hours could have gone somewhere they would have mattered more.

The mistakes are not the point. They happen. They are part of the deal. The point is to do less of them, and to forgive yourself for the ones you make.

Things I Did Right

It's worth saying these too. Not to brag — these are just the choices I'm grateful I made. If any of them help you make a similar one, good.

- **I kept our families close.** Friday night dinners with Dave's cousin and his wife. Having his brother and sister-in-law over. Small, ordinary nights — the kind you don't think you'll remember. We remember them.
- **I made room for Dave and his mother.** They had a close relationship — he loved her dearly — and whatever else was happening that week, I tried not to let that get crowded out.
- **I told my son the truth.** He was four. I prepared him for losing his father in language he could understand. After Dave was gone, I got him into therapy. It is a hard thing to be that young and

lose a parent. I didn't want him to have to carry it alone.

- **I made Dave have the hard conversations.** The nurse in me knew we needed them. I knew what his wishes were before we had to act on them. When he said he was done, I honored that. So often, our loved ones suffer longer than they want to because the people around them aren't ready to let them go. I didn't want that for him.

What Actually Matters

After everything — after all the chapters and the checklists and the scripts and the systems — here is what I think actually matters most. The short list. The one I'd save.

- **Showing up.** Not perfectly. Just consistently. Being there is most of it.
- **Listening.** To your loved one. To the team. To your own gut.
- **Asking the question.** When in doubt, out loud.
- **Documenting.** It saves you. It saves them.
- **Advocating.** Calmly, persistently, specifically. The job no one else is going to do.
- **Honoring their wishes.** Once they tell you what they want, do everything you can to make it that way.
- **Taking care of yourself.** Bare minimum survival. Sleep, water, food, sun, one human.
- **Forgiving yourself.** Often.
- **Letting people in.** The ones who show up. Let them. You don't have to do this alone.
- **Letting yourself cry.** You'll need it. When you're done, you'll feel a little better. That is allowed.
- **Saying the things.** "I love you." "Thank you." "I'm sorry." "I forgive you." "You matter to me." Don't save them for the last week.
- **Telling them it's okay to go.** When you're at the end, it is okay to say it out loud. That you'll miss them. That you'll be okay.

That you'll love them, always. Sometimes they need to hear it before they can leave.

* * *

Toward the end, Dave's behavior started shifting. Subtle at first, then not. On April 1st, I made him go to the ED. I had fought too hard to keep him alive — I was not letting him go from a stroke. They kept him overnight, did a PET scan the next morning, and that's when we found out. The CNS lymphoma was back. With a vengeance.

He told me he was done. No more five-day admissions for high-dose methotrexate. He wanted to go on his terms.

We had agreed, all along, that we'd fight as long as he wanted to fight. When he was tired, we'd talk. This was that talk. I supported him.

That Saturday, his words came out jumbled. He couldn't get them where he wanted them to go, and it frustrated the hell out of him. Hell, it frustrated me too. I was in the shower — where all great ideas come from — when I got the gut instinct to take him to camp. The place he loved. The place where the extended family always ended up. Pizza and a fire.

I didn't ask Dave first. I called his cousin and told him, "I need your help. We're going to camp tonight. Round up whoever you can." Once the plans were locked in, I told Dave. I expected him to push back. He didn't.

We took his truck — his newest baby. A 2023 Ford F-150 Krietz Custom. Lifted. Beautiful. He'd bought it the October before. On the way to camp, his window was down, and I went to roll it up. The look he gave me said no. I asked, "Do you want it down?" He nodded and rolled it back down himself.

I reached over and grabbed his hand. "Am I doing the right thing? Making you go out here?"

He turned to me. Smiled. Nodded. Squeezed my hand.

That night, his family and friends got to drink a beer with Dave, in a place we all loved, one last time.

* * *

A Word to the Caregiver Reading This Late at Night

If you are reading this at 2 a.m. with a sleeping person down the hall and a notebook full of questions and a heart that is too full and too empty at the same time — I see you.

I know what you carry. I know how invisible most of it is. I know the loneliness of being the person everyone expects to handle this. I know the silence after a hard day.

You are doing one of the most important things a human being can do. Not in a dramatic way. In the quiet, daily, exhausting way. By showing up. By asking the questions. By holding their hand. By making the calls. By not giving up when the system tries to wear you down.

It will not feel like enough most days. It is enough. You are enough.

You are not alone. There are millions of us, somewhere out there in the dark, doing the same thing. We see each other, even when nobody else does.

* * *

Do This Next

- **Read this chapter again on a hard day.** This is the one to come back to.
- **Write your own list.** What do you wish you'd known at the beginning? Even if you're still in the middle, you've learned things. Write them down. Future you, or future them, will need them.
- **If you read one thing from this whole book and didn't act on it, do that one thing now.** Make the call. Print the list. Have the conversation. Sign the paperwork. The book is only as useful as what

you do with it.

- **Take a moment of credit for being here.** You picked up this book. You read this far. You are doing the work. That counts. Don't let yourself talk you out of it.

* * *

One more section after this: the toolbox. Checklists, scripts, worksheets, quick references. The pull-it-out-and-use-it stuff. Print what helps. Skip what doesn't. This whole book exists to make your job easier. Use it like a tool.

And take care of yourself. I mean it.

With you in this always,

Tiffany

Bonus Section: Tools & Resources

The Pull-It-Out-and-Use-It Stuff

This section is the toolbox. Checklists, worksheets, scripts, and quick-reference guides. Print what helps. Tape it to the fridge. Stick it in your binder. This isn't meant to be read straight through — it's meant to be grabbed in a moment when you need it.

* * *

Caregiver Day-One Checklist

If you're at the very beginning, do these first.

- Get a notebook. Label it. Carry it.
- Take photos of the insurance card (front and back).
- Set up the patient portal.
- Sign a HIPAA release at the next visit.
- Start the medication list.
- Build the contact list (PCP, specialists, pharmacy, case manag-

er).

- Get a power of attorney for healthcare in place if possible.
- Pick a system for organizing (binder, phone folder, hybrid).
- Identify one person to share information with.

Go-In-With-This Appointment Checklist

- Photo ID and insurance card
- Updated medication list (printed)
- Symptom timeline / what's changed since last visit
- Top 3 questions written down
- List of other doctors involved + recent procedures or hospitalizations
- Pen and notebook (or phone with notes app open)
- Referral or authorization confirmation, if relevant
- Recent lab/imaging reports if seeing a new provider
- HIPAA release filed at this office

Hospital Stay Daily Ask Checklist

Ask these every day:

- What changed in the last 24 hours, for better or worse?
- What is the working diagnosis right now?
- What are we doing today and tomorrow?
- What are the criteria for discharge?
- What is the estimated discharge date?
- Where will [patient] go after discharge?
- What questions should I bring up with the team today?

Discharge Checklist (Before Leaving the Hospital)

☐ Discharge summary received and read

☐ All medications reconciled (home list vs new list)

☐ New prescriptions sent to pharmacy

☐ Any equipment/oxygen/home health arranged

☐ Follow-up appointments scheduled (PCP, specialists)

☐ Warning signs / when to call clearly written down

☐ Phone numbers to call if something goes wrong overnight

☐ Case manager contact info

☐ Inpatient vs observation status confirmed (if going to SNF)

Hospice Transition Checklist

For the day or week when hospice becomes the conversation. Use it to keep your head while everything is moving.

Before You Decide

☐ Confirm the doctor's prognosis: terminal, six months or less

☐ Ask if a bridge program or palliative care exists if you're not ready for full hospice

☐ Talk to your loved one. What do they want? Listen.

☐ Get the family on the same page — or at least informed

Choosing a Hospice

☐ Ask the hospital case manager for options in your area

☐ Check Medicare.gov's Hospice Compare tool for ratings

☐ Ask about: 24/7 on-call nurse, visit frequency, social work, chaplain, bereavement support

☐ Ask about respite care (short stays so you can rest)

☐ Ask about the four levels of care: routine, continuous, inpatient, respite

Where Will They Be

☐ At home (most people)

☐ At a hospice house

☐ In a nursing facility with hospice services

☐ In a hospital, for short-term symptom management

Paperwork to Have in Place

☐ Healthcare power of attorney

☐ Advance directive

☐ DNR (Do Not Resuscitate), if appropriate

☐ POLST or MOLST (varies by state)

☐ Funeral home selected (it sounds early; it's not)

Day-One Questions for the Hospice Team

☐ Who is our primary nurse, and how do I reach them after hours?

☐ What medications will be in the house — what's each one for?

☐ What equipment is coming, and when?

☐ When do I call you, and when do I call 911?

☐ What does the bereavement program look like for our family?

Checklists to Care for You!

Hospital Bag for the Caregiver

- Phone charger + extra-long cable
- Charging brick (battery pack)
- Sweater or zip-up (ICUs are cold)
- Reusable water bottle
- Snacks (protein bars, nuts)
- Medication list and insurance card photos
- Notebook and two pens
- Headphones
- Toothbrush and small toiletries
- Cash in small bills (vending machines, parking)
- Glasses, hearing aids, dentures (for the patient)
- List of questions you want to ask the team

Bare Minimum Survival Day Checklist

☐ Got dressed (real clothes)

☐ Ate three times

☐ Drank water

☐ Stepped outside once

☐ Talked to one safe person

☐ Will sleep tonight

After It's Over Checklist

The first weeks after loss are a fog. This is the list nobody hands you. Do what you can, when you can.

Right Away (Immediately Through the First Week)

☐ Order at least 10 certified copies of the death certificate (you'll need more than you think)

☐ Notify the funeral home — they often handle Social Security notification and the obituary

☐ Call close family and friends, or ask one person to make the calls for you

☐ Notify employer if your loved one was working

☐ Locate the will, if there is one — and there should be one, since we covered this earlier. Having one makes everything easier.

☐ Secure the home, vehicles, and any pets

In the First Month

☐ Notify Social Security (often done by funeral home)

☐ Notify life insurance — start the claim

☐ Notify health insurance to end coverage

☐ Notify pension or retirement plan administrators

☐ Notify the VA, if your loved one was a veteran

☐ Notify the mortgage company or landlord

☐ Notify the auto loan or lease company

☐ Update beneficiaries on your own accounts

☐ Stop or transfer subscriptions and memberships

☐ Close or transfer credit cards in your loved one's name only

☐ If filing taxes jointly, talk to a tax professional

In the First Year

☐ Don't make major life decisions if you can avoid it (selling the house, big moves, big purchases)

☐ See your own doctor when you have the energy

☐ Find a grief resource that fits — therapist, group, church, walks

☐ Pick one person to be your call buddy for the paperwork days

☐ On the hard days, read Chapter 18 again

If You Have Children

☐ Get them into therapy. Even if they seem fine.

☐ Tell their school. Their teachers need to know.

☐ Be honest, in language they can understand.

☐ Talk about the parent who died often. Don't make their name a forbidden word.

* * *

Worksheet: Know Your Insurance

Sit with the insurance card and summary of benefits. Fill in the answers.

- Insurance company name: ___________
- Plan name: ___________
- Plan type (HMO, PPO, EPO, Medicare Advantage, etc.) : ___________
- Member ID: ___________
- Group number: ___________
- Customer service phone (back of card): ___________
- Annual deductible (in-network): $___________
- Annual out-of-pocket maximum (in-network): $___________
- Coinsurance percentage (in-network): ___________

- PCP copay: $__________
- Specialist copay: $__________
- ER copay: $__________
- Urgent care copay: $__________
- Does this plan require referrals? Yes / No
- Where do I check authorization status? __________
- Plan year: __________

Worksheet: Master Medication List

One row per medication. Update with every change.

- Drug name (brand / generic): __________
- Dose: __________
- Frequency: __________
- Route (mouth, injection, etc.): __________
- What it's for (plain English): __________
- Prescribed by: __________
- Start date: __________

Don't forget OTC medications, vitamins, and supplements.

Allergies and reactions: __________

Worksheet: Medical History One-Pager

- Patient name: __________
- Date of birth: __________
- PCP name and phone: __________
- Active diagnoses (with year): __________
- Major surgeries (year, hospital, what was done): __________
- Allergies and reactions: __________
- Implanted devices: __________
- Recent hospitalizations (last 12 months): __________
- Code status / advance directive in place: __________

- Healthcare power of attorney name and phone: __________

Worksheet: What Your Loved One Wants

Have the conversation while you can. Fill it in together if they want to. Skip the parts that don't apply.

Where do you want to be at the end?

☐ At home

☐ At a hospice house

☐ In a hospital, if needed

☐ No preference

Who do you want with you?

- Specific names: __________

☐ As many people as want to be there

☐ Just immediate family

☐ No preference

Medically, what do you want?

☐ Aggressive treatment as long as possible

☐ Comfort care only when [milestone — e.g., "I can't recognize my children"]

☐ Switch to hospice if doctors estimate six months or less

- DNR (do not resuscitate): yes / no
- Feeding tube: yes / no / only if temporary
- Ventilator: yes / no / only if temporary

Funeral / memorial preferences:

- Burial / Cremation (circle one)
- Funeral home: __________
- Cemetery or scattering location: __________
- Service style: religious / non-religious / celebration of life / private / public
- Songs, readings, speakers: __________

- Obituary preferences: __________

What do you want your loved ones to know?

____

____

Anyone you want NOT involved? (It's okay to say so.)

____

This is a starting point, not a script. Have the conversation. Write things down. Update as wishes change.

Worksheet: Healthcare Contacts

One row per provider/contact. Format example:

Dr. Sarah Chen — Cardiologist — Heartwell Clinic — (555) 123-4567 — fax (555) 123-4570 — manages: heart failure meds

- PCP: __________
- Specialists: __________
- Preferred pharmacy: __________
- Case manager: __________
- Home health agency: __________
- DME (durable medical equipment) supplier: __________
- Hospice (if applicable): __________

Worksheet: Authorization Tracker

Track every prior authorization or referral. One row per request.

- Date ordered: __________
- Service ordered: __________
- Provider who ordered: __________
- Date submitted to insurance: __________
- Status: Pending / Approved / Denied
- Reference number: __________
- Date of last follow-up call: __________

- Person spoken with: __________
- Next step: __________

Worksheet: Bill Tracker

Track every bill and EOB.

- Date of service: __________
- Provider/facility: __________
- Amount charged: __________
- Amount allowed (per EOB): __________
- Insurance paid: __________
- Patient responsibility: __________
- Bill received? Date: __________
- Paid? Date / amount: __________
- Notes (questions, disputes): __________

Worksheet: Help-Wanted List

When someone asks, "What can I do to help?" — pull from this list.

- Bring a meal
- Sit with [my person] for an hour
- Take [my person] to one appointment
- Grocery run
- Pick up the kids from school
- Mow the lawn / shovel the driveway
- Drop off coffee at the hospital
- Make a specific phone call I'm dreading
- Sit with me at chemo / dialysis / appointment
- Just text me randomly to check on me

* * *

Talking to Kids About a Dying Parent

The hardest conversation, with the most important person. Here is what helps. None of it makes it easy. All of it is better than silence.

Use real words.

"Dying," "died," "death." Not "passed away," "lost," "gone to sleep," "with the angels." Children take words literally. "Lost" makes them think the person can be found. "Sleep" makes them afraid of bedtime. Real words, gently said, let them understand what is actually happening.

Match their age.

- **Under 5:** simple and concrete. "Daddy is very, very sick. The doctors can't fix it. His body is going to stop working, and he is going to die."
- **5 to 9:** a little more detail. Expect questions about the body — where it goes, what happens to it. Answer factually.
- **10 to 12:** they grasp permanence. They may go quiet, or get angry. Both are normal.
- **Teens:** emotionally like adults, with less life experience. They need information, and space to react.

Answer the question they actually asked.

Not the one you think they meant.

- **"Are you going to die too?"** — "Not for a very long time, I hope. I'm healthy. And if anything ever happened to me, [list of people] would take care of you."
- **"Did I cause this?"** — "No. Nothing you did, said, or thought caused this."

Don't promise things you can't keep.

"Nothing bad will ever happen to me" is a promise you can't make. Try: "I'm healthy. I plan to be here for a very long time."

After the death.

- Tell their school immediately. The teacher should know before the child is back in class.

- Get them into therapy. Even if they seem fine. Especially if they seem fine.
- Keep talking about the parent who died. Use their name. Look at photos. Say "Daddy would have loved this."
- Watch for delayed grief. It can show up months later as anger, school issues, or sudden tears.

Resources for grieving kids are at the end of this section.

* * *

Scripts for Difficult Conversations

Calling the Provider's Office About a PA

"Hi, this is [your name] calling for [patient name], DOB [date]. Dr. [name] ordered [procedure] on [date]. I'm calling to check on the prior authorization. Can you tell me whether it's been submitted, and if so, the status?"

Calling Insurance Member Services

"Hi, I'm calling on behalf of [patient name], member ID [#], DOB [date]. There's a prior authorization request from Dr. [name]'s office for [procedure], submitted on [date]. Can you tell me the status, and if there's any missing information?"

When You Don't Understand

"I need clarification on what you just said. Can you explain it again — maybe in plainer language?"

When You Want the Reasoning

"Can you walk me through why we're choosing this approach over another option?"

When Something Feels Off

"I may be missing something, but I'm noticing [specific observation]. Can the team take another look?"

When Being Brushed Off

"I'd like to be sure this is documented. Can you note in the chart that I asked about [specific concern]?"

When You Need More Time to Decide

"Before we make this decision, I'd like a few minutes to talk it through with my family. Can we have 15 minutes?"

When You Want to Slow Down a Discharge

"I'm worried she's not stable enough to leave today. Can we talk about what would need to be in place for her to be discharged safely?"

Asking About Hospice

"Are we at a point where we should be thinking about hospice or comfort-focused care?"

Asking About Time

"What is your best guess about how much time we have, in terms of months, weeks, or days?"

Starting the Hard Conversation With Your Loved One

"I know we don't usually talk about this. I want to make sure that if something happens, I'm able to make decisions the way you would want them made. Can we talk about what matters to you?"

Calling Billing About a Bill

"Hi, I'm calling about a bill for [patient name], account number [#], date of service [date]. The amount is $[X]. I'm trying to understand the charges — can you walk me through them, and confirm whether insurance has finished processing?"

Asking for a Self-Pay Discount

"If I were able to pay this in a lump sum, what discount could you offer?"

Asking for Financial Assistance

"I received a bill for $[X]. I don't have the means to pay this in full. Do you have a financial assistance program, and can you send me the

application?"

Setting a Boundary With a Critical Family Member

"I'm doing my best. I'm not going to keep talking about whether I'm doing it right with someone who isn't here. If you'd like to help, I'd love that."

Asking for Specific Help

"Yes — could you sit with [my person] for an hour Saturday so I can take a walk?"

Telling Them It's Okay to Go

"I love you. I'm going to miss you so much. But I'm going to be okay. The kids are going to be okay. You don't have to hold on for us. It's okay to go when you're ready."

Calling 911 With Hospice in Place

If you or family panic and need EMS — lead with this.

"I'm calling about [patient name], DOB [date]. They are on hospice with [hospice agency]. The hospice nurse is [name], number [phone]. Comfort measures only — no resuscitation. Please contact the hospice on-call line before sending units."

Note: Most hospice deaths do not need EMS. Call your hospice on-call line first. EMS is for: an emergency hospice can't manage at home, or family that wants help and can't reach hospice.

* * *

Quick-Reference Guides

Where to Go: Primary Care vs Urgent Care vs ER

- **Could die or be permanently harmed in next few hours** — ER. Call 911 if appropriate.
- **Annoying but not dangerous** — urgent care.
- **Ongoing or routine** — primary care.
- **When in doubt** — default up.

Stroke Signs (FAST)

- **F**ace drooping
- **A**rm weakness
- **S**peech difficulty
- **T**ime to call 911

Always Call 911 For

- Chest pain or pressure (especially with shortness of breath, nausea, sweating)
- Stroke signs
- Severe difficulty breathing
- Loss of consciousness
- Severe injury or major bleeding
- Suspected overdose
- New severe confusion in an elderly person
- Fall in someone on blood thinners (even if they "seem fine")

Who to Call When

- **Question about a medication** — pharmacist or prescribing provider
- **New non-emergency symptom** — PCP office during business hours
- **Trouble getting an authorization** — provider's office first, then insurance
- **Question about a bill** — billing department on the bill
- **Question about coverage** — member services on the back of the card
- **Hospital admission, discharge, rehab placement** — case manager
- **Concern about hospital floor care** — bedside nurse — charge nurse — supervisor
- **Mental health crisis** — 988 or 911

Chain of Command (Hospital)

- Bedside nurse
- Charge nurse
- Nursing supervisor
- Director of Nursing
- Chief Nursing Officer
- Hospitalist or attending physician
- Patient advocate / patient relations
- Rapid response team (for acute clinical concerns; ask if your hospital has one)
- Hospital ethics committee (for genuinely complex disagreements about care)

Chain of Command (Insurance)

- Member services rep
- Supervisor
- Case management at the insurer
- Formal grievance / complaint
- State insurance commissioner

Insurance Terms in 60 Seconds

- **Premium** — monthly cost to have the plan.
- **Deductible** — amount you pay before insurance kicks in.
- **Coinsurance** — percentage you pay after deductible (e.g., 20%).
- **Copay** — flat fee at time of service.
- **Out-of-pocket max** — most you'll pay in a year for covered services.
- **Referral** — PCP saying yes to a specialist visit.
- **Prior authorization (PA)** — insurance saying yes to a specific service.
- **EOB (Explanation of Benefits)** — NOT a bill. Summary of

what insurance did.

- **Bill** — actual statement asking for payment.

Bill vs EOB Cheat Sheet

- **EOB** comes from insurance. Says "THIS IS NOT A BILL." Wait for it before paying anything.
- **Bill** comes from provider. Compare to EOB. If amounts don't match, call billing.
- **Don't pay until** the EOB has come and you've compared.

Appeal Timeline (Standard)

- **Deadline to file appeal:** typically 60–180 days from denial — check the letter.
- **Insurer response time:** typically 30 days standard, 72 hours expedited.
- **Levels of appeal:** internal (1–2 levels) — external review.

Hospice vs Palliative Care

- **Palliative care** = comfort/symptom care alongside any treatment, at any stage of serious illness.
- **Hospice** = comfort care for people whose physician estimates 6 months or less. Active treatment for the terminal disease typically stops; comfort care is the focus.

Daily Caregiver Reminders

Eat. Drink. Sleep. Move. Sun. One human.

* * *

Resources Worth Knowing

- **Medicare.gov** — official Medicare site, including claims and appeals walkthroughs.
- **SHIP (State Health Insurance Assistance Program)** — free Medicare counseling, every state.
- **Family Caregiver Alliance (caregiver.org)** — caregiver sup-

port, resources, by state.

- **Eldercare Locator (eldercare.acl.gov, 1-800-677-1116)** — federal directory of services for older adults.
- **National Hospice and Palliative Care Organization (nhpco.org)** — info on hospice and how to find a provider.
- **988 Suicide and Crisis Lifeline** — call or text.
- **Long-term care ombudsman (ltcombudsman.org)** — advocates for residents of long-term care facilities, every state.
- **No Surprises Act resources** — cms.gov/nosurprises for surprise billing protections.
- **Healthcare Bluebook / FAIR Health Consumer** — estimate fair prices for medical services.
- **GoodRx / SingleCare** — prescription discount programs.
- **Patient assistance programs** — most expensive medications have manufacturer programs (Google "[drug name] patient assistance").
- **State insurance commissioner** — file complaints about insurer behavior; search "[your state] insurance commissioner."

For Grieving Kids

- **The Dougy Center (dougy.org)** — national leader in children's grief support, with local chapters and free guides.
- **National Alliance for Children's Grief (childrengrieve.org)** — find a local children's grief program.
- **Sesame Street in Communities (sesamestreetincommunities.org)** — free grief videos and tools for young kids, co-developed with grief experts.
- **Comfort Zone Camp (comfortzonecamp.org)** — free bereavement camps for kids who lost a parent or sibling.
- **Your local children's hospital** — most have a bereavement program, often free, even if your child was never a patient.

- **The school counselor** — start there if you can't find anything else; they can connect you to local resources.

* * *

A Final Word

This whole book is meant to make your job a little less impossible. Rip pages out. Highlight what matters. Ignore what doesn't apply. Use it like a tool, not like scripture.

If even one chapter saves you a phone call, a sleepless night, or a misunderstanding — it's done its job.

And if it didn't — thank you for trying. You're doing more than you know.

Take care of yourself. I mean it.

—

With you in this always,

Tiffany

Acknowledgements

No book like this gets written alone, and there are people I need to thank.

To my husband, Dave — though you are no longer with us on this earth, I know you are with me always. You gave me the strength I needed to write this book, to help others.

To my son, Finnegan — always remember that your daddy loved you so very much.

And to WV Caring — the care you provided to both Dave and my Mom-mom Brenda was top of the line. We could not have handled everything we did, in such a short amount of time, without you.

To all the family and friends I did not mention, I am sorry, but I get charged per print page and I cannot afford a 200-page acknowledgement. Just know that I love you.

To every reader who picked up this book — thank you. I hope it helps.

— Tiffany

About the Author

I'm Tiffany Auvil — a nurse, a caregiver, a widow, and a mom.

I've been a nurse for twenty years. I started as an LPN in 2005, spent my first three years in bedside nursing, and then moved into ambulatory care, where I spent most of my career. I became an RN in 2022 and earned my MBA in Healthcare Administration in January 2026. I'm currently enrolled in the Doctor of Science in Integrative Healthcare program at the American College of Healthcare Sciences. I'm a lifelong learner. School and courses are some of the few things that have always made sense to me.

But none of that is what made me write this book.

This book exists because of Dave.

I cared for my husband from January 2023 until he died in April 2025. His original diagnosis was renal cell carcinoma that metastasized to his liver and pancreas. Then, in February 2024, he was diagnosed with a second, separate cancer — a CNS lymphoma. Two different cancers, at the same time, in the same person. The two and a half years between his first diagnosis and his death were the hardest, most clarifying time of my life.

I knew the healthcare system. I'd spent two decades inside it. And it still nearly broke me. There was a moment when a clerical error almost delayed Dave's immunotherapy — and if it had, we would have lost him months sooner than we did. I remember thinking: *I caught that because I knew where to look. How many families don't? How many people are losing time, or losing the people they love, because nobody told them how the system actually works?*

That question is the reason this book exists.

I live in Parsons, West Virginia, with my five-year-old son, Finnegan, and the rest of our chaos: Quill the dog, Groot and Damian the cats (Groot was Dave's; he tolerates me now), Rocket the gecko, and Yondu the hermit crab. Parsons is a small town with a big heart, and it lived up to that during Dave's illness in a way I'll never forget. The night of his viewing, I stood by his casket for three hours straight. The line never broke. People I hadn't seen in years came to hug me, to say goodbye to Dave, to bring Finnegan a present. Dave used to say nobody would come to his funeral. He was wrong about that. He was wrong about a lot of things in the best way.

When I'm not raising Finnegan or working on my doctorate, I'm usually crafting — resin work, knitting, crocheting when I have the patience. On warm days, you'll find me in the river hunting for rocks. And if I'm lucky enough to get to the beach on vacation, I'll be hunting for seashells. I'm trying to build a life where I can be of service to caregivers, because I think the people doing this work deserve more than what the system gives them.

This is my first book. It will not be my last.

You can find me at **www.tiffanyauvil.com**, on Facebook as Tiffany Curran Auvil, on LinkedIn as Tiffany Auvil, or by email at **tiffany@tiffanyauvil.com**. If this book helped you, I'd love to hear about it. If it didn't, I'd love to hear about that too.

— Tiffany

www.ingramcontent.com/pod-product-compliance
Ingram Content Group UK Ltd.
Pitfield, Milton Keynes, MK11 3LW, UK
UKHW041954190726
13854UKWH00005B/1972

9 798996 088225